OXFORD MEDICAL PUBLICATIONS

Stroke care

Stroke care: a practical manual

Rowan H. Harwood

Consultant Physician & Geriatrician
City Hospital, Nottingham, UK

Farhad Huwez

Consultant physician/Stroke Services
Basildon Hospital, Essex, UK

Dawn Good

Clinical Stroke Service Specialist
City Hospital, Nottingham, UK

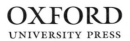

OXFORD
UNIVERSITY PRESS

OXFORD
UNIVERSITY PRESS

Great Clarendon Street, Oxford OX2 6DP

Oxford University Press is a department of the University of Oxford.
It furthers the University's objective of excellence in research, scholarship,
and education by publishing worldwide in

Oxford New York

Auckland Cape Town Dar es Salaam Hong Kong Karachi
Kuala Lumpur Madrid Melbourne Mexico City Nairobi
New Delhi Shanghai Taipei Toronto

With offices in

Argentina Austria Brazil Chile Czech Republic France Greece
Guatemala Hungary Italy Japan South Korea Poland Portugal
Singapore Switzerland Thailand Turkey Ukraine Vietnam

Oxford is a registered trade mark of Oxford University Press
in the UK and in certain other countries

Published in the United States
by Oxford University Press Inc., New York

A catalogue record for this title is available from the British Library

Library of Congress Cataloging in Publication Data

Harwood, Rowan.
Oxford handbook of stroke care : a practical manual / Rowan H. Harwood, Farhad
Huwez, Dawn Good.
Includes bibliographical references and index.
1. Cerebrovascular disease–Handbooks, manuals, etc.
[DNLM: 1. Cerebrovascular Accident—therapy—Handbooks. WL 39 H343o 2005] I.
Title: Handbook of stroke care. II. Title: Stroke care. III. Huwez, Farhad. IV. Good,
Dawn. V. Oxford University Press. VI. Title.
RC388.5.H37 2005   616.8'1—dc22   2004024497

ISBN 0 19 852973 2 (Pbk. : alk. paper)

10 9 8 7 6 5 4 3 2 1

Typeset by Newgen Imaging Systems (P) Ltd., Chennai, India
Printed in Italy
on acid-free paper by Grafiche Industriali

Preface

This book is written for people who look after stroke patients, in particular, doctors and nurses working in hospitals. A new staff member, or a doctor rotating onto the stroke unit, may find it useful to read through the book, but this is also a book to refer back to.

We aim to give practical advice. We are well aware of the need to justify bold assertions with high-quality evidence. The quality of the evidence we have available is variable. Statements that lack the backing of a RCT are both uncertain to some extent, and vulnerable to change as new findings emerge. If you want a catalogue of RCT evidence, however, other resources exist, such as the Cochrane Library. Moreover, the RCT is not the only type of evidence. The applicability of a given RCT result may be open to question, when faced with the particular circumstances of the patient in front of you. Sometimes decisions have to be made in the absence of RCT guidance. Much of our advice is based on experience, or what we have been taught, illuminated by hard evidence where it is available, or where sensible extrapolations can be made from what is known.

Our main text is, perhaps, a little dogmatic. If you are faced with a problem, you need to know what do. You might want to follow-up the evidence for what we suggest, but that is not our main purpose. We present key pieces of evidence in a fairly raw form in boxes scattered throughout the text. We confine references to these boxes. We doubt that any more would be used much, and there are more encyclopaedic reference texts or electronic searching with which we are not trying to compete.

We follow a time-based sequence of chapters, which follows the journey of a stroke patient from diagnosis to outcomes. We take a very broad view of what stroke care requires. We are writing from the perspective of general internal and geriatric medicine rather than as specialist neurologists. We struggle most when working at the limits of our knowledge and experience. In this book we push at the boundaries of the subject. For example, the quality of clinical decision making is very topical, has made an appearance in some postgraduate examinations, and we spend large amounts of clinical time working on difficult decisions. Therefore, we include a chapter on it. Many stroke patients die, so we include a chapter on terminal care. Advice on managing undiagnosed coma, pain, and disturbed behaviour are not specific to stroke, but are all situations that have arisen in our own stroke practices.

There is some repetition. Some issues arise early and persist (such as positioning, venous thrombosis prophylaxis, and continence). The distinction between acute and rehabilitation care is blurred. Secondary prevention can often start quite early rather than the end of the process as our chapter order suggests. Hopefully any repetition makes each section more self-contained than it would otherwise be.

This is a book of guidelines. Guidelines are intended to give help and advice, but are not a substitute for proper professional assessment and opinion. Evidence changes with time, interpretation of evidence may vary with circumstances and from individual to individual, and different places have quite justifiably different ways of doing things. We have checked drug doses, but correct prescription remains the responsibility of the prescriber, who may need to take account of local policies or guidelines. Similarly, on legal and ethical issues, we write from the perspective of the law and current practice in England and Wales, but hope that the general principles will be of interest and use elsewhere.

We have taken advice from a large number of people in writing this book, including Peter Berman, Vincent Crosby, Leela Duari, John Gladman, Tony Goddard, Suzanne Hawkins, Miles Humberstone, Tim Jaspan, Roger Knaggs, Charlotte Morton, Jan Riley, Nina Squires, Udayaraj UmaSankar, and Mark Willmot. We are very grateful to them. Mistakes are our own.

We must also thank our patients and their families, who inspired us to look at stroke medicine as a 'defined speciality', requiring organized care by a team that has interest and expertise. We would like to dedicate this book to them.

RH
FH
DG

Contents

Abbreviations

ACE	angiotensin converting enzyme
ACEI	angiotensin converting enzyme inhibitors
ADH	antidiuretic hormone
APTT	activated partial thromboplastin time
bd	twice a day
BP	blood pressure
CAST	Chinese Acute Stroke Trial
CCB	calcium channel blocker
CI	confidence interval
CPR	cardiopulmonary resuscitation
CSF	cerebrospinal fluid
CT	computed tomography
CTA	computed tomographic angiography
DNR	do not resuscitate
DVT	deep vein thrombosis
ECASS	European Co-operative Acute Stroke Study
ECG	electrocardiogram/electrocardiography
ESR	erythrocyte sedimentation rate
FBC	full blood count
IM	intramuscular
INR	international normalized ratio (for warfarin anticoagulation control)
ISAT	International Subarachnoid Aneurysm Trial
IST	International Stroke Trial
ITT	intention-to-treat
IV	intravenous
LACI	lacunar infarct
LMWH	low molecular weight heparin
MI	myocardial infarction
MMSE	Mini-Mental State Examination
MRA	magnetic resonance angiography
MRI	magnetic resonance imaging
NHS	National Health Service
NINDS	National Institute of Neurological Disorders and Stroke
NNT	numbers needed to treat

OCSP	Oxfordshire Community Stroke Project
od	once a day
OR	odds ratio
OT	occupational therapist
PACI	partial anterior circulation infarct
PEG	percutaneous endoscopic gastrostomy
POCI	posterior circulation infarct
qds	to be taken four times a day
RCT	randomized controlled trial
RR	relative risk
SAH	subarachnoid haemorrhage
SC	subcutaneous
SIADH	syndrome of inappropriate antidiuretic hormone secretion
SSS	Scandinavian Stroke Score
TACI	total anterior circulation infarct
tds	to be taken three times a day
TIA	transient ischaemic attack
tPA	tissue plasminogen activator
vs.	versus
WFNS	World Federation of Neurological Surgeons

Chapter 1

Is it a stroke?

Presentation of stroke

A diagnosis is an explanation, in biological terms, of a problem that a patient presents. An accurate diagnosis allows you to:

- Initiate specific treatments (and avoid worthless ones).
- Give an explanation of what is going on to the patient and others.
- Indicate chances of recovery and recurrence.

Many subsequent management decisions (medical, nursing, and rehabilitation) assume that the working diagnosis is correct.

Stroke is a syndrome—a collection of symptoms and signs, which are usually obvious. It is defined as:

a rapidly developing episode of focal or global neurological dysfunction, lasting longer than 24 h or leading to death, and of presumed vascular origin.

This definition is reasonable for many purposes, but has limitations:

- Some patients who appear to have had a stroke, have something other than cerebral infarction or haemorrhage (sometimes called 'stroke-mimics').
- Neurological deficit progresses to some extent over the first 24 h in about 25% of cases, and secondary deterioration within the first week is common.
- It tells us nothing about the underlying pathology. More precise characterization of the type of stroke gives us clues about treatment options, prognosis, and risk of recurrence.
- Some non-specific presentations (immobility, falls, confusion, or incontinence) may be due to vascular brain disease, among other things.
- Comorbid conditions (especially in elderly people) can make diagnosis difficult.
- A number of cerebrovascular conditions fall outside the definition, including vascular dementia, silent infarction on brain imaging, and TIA.
- SAH fits the clinical definition for a stroke, but behaves and is managed as a separate entity.

What else might it be?

Transient ischaemic attack

- A TIA is an acute loss of focal cerebral function, or transient monocular blindness (amaurosis fugax), of presumed vascular origin, but the symptoms last less than 24 h.
- Initially it is indistinguishable from a stroke.
- Most TIAs last less than an hour.
- Amaurosis fugax is a rapidly progressive loss of vision in one eye (often, but not exclusively, 'like a curtain coming down'), coming on over a few seconds to a minute. After a variable time, usually only a few minutes, it resolves with gradual recovery of vision over the whole visual field.
- Hemiplegic migraine is excluded.
- The main difficulty is making an accurate diagnosis based only on the history, and the absence of examination or investigation findings that suggest another diagnosis.
- Patients with TIA and minor stroke should be offered thorough investigation, and appropriate secondary prevention.
- Risk factors, and prognosis for stroke recurrence and ischaemic heart disease, are identical for TIA and minor stroke, regardless of symptom duration.
- About a quarter of patients with clinical TIA have an appropriate infarct on brain imaging (more on diffusion-weighted magnetic resonance images).
- Transient dizziness, confusion, vertigo, double vision, syncope, and drop attacks should not be diagnosed as TIA in the absence of other neurological findings.
- If thrombolysis is being considered for acute stroke, treatment must be delivered within 3 h of symptom onset. Work-up must therefore begin without waiting to see if the deficit will resolve spontaneously; although in the face of rapidly resolving symptoms administering potentially dangerous treatment would be unwise.

Other differential diagnoses

- From the perspective of hospital admissions, 10–20% of patients referred with possible stroke have something else.
- Some uncertainty is inevitable, but experienced doctors are better at diagnosing (and ruling out) stroke than less experienced ones.
- Important differential diagnoses are shown in Table 1.1. Others that sometimes arise include psychiatric illnesses, multiple sclerosis, metabolic disturbances, intoxication, transient global amnesia, dementia, and Parkinson's disease.
- Ask a neurologist's opinion if you are struggling to explain the clinical features, or are considering some of the more difficult or rare diagnoses.

Table 1.1 Conditions that can cause stroke-syndrome ('stroke-mimics')

Diagnosis	Key features
Fits, with Todd's paresis	Commonest cause for misdiagnosis of recurrent stroke. Clinical diagnosis, usually requiring an eyewitness. Consider ictal features (loss of consciousness, convulsions, tongue biting, incontinence) and postictal features (headache, sleepiness, confusion).
Cerebral tumours, primary or secondary	CT scan diagnosis. There may be features of raised intracranial pressure (headache, vomiting, drowsiness, papilloedema). Onset is slower than stroke. A step-wise progression over days or weeks is associated with space-occupying lesions, but only 1 in 6 patients with a progressive course has a tumour. Onset may be sudden if there is bleeding into a tumour.
Hypoglycaemia	Almost always drug-induced, severe, hypoglycaemia. Usually rapidly reversible, but hemiplegia can persist 24 h or more.
Subdural haematoma	CT scan diagnosis. If significant, will cause drowsiness. Sometimes headache, confusion, hemiplegia, or dysphasia. Features may fluctuate.
Cerebral abscess	CT scan diagnosis. Usually due to spread from sinuses or ear. Onset is subacute, but there are not always prodromal infective symptoms. Headache usual. Later drowsiness, vomiting, delirium, and bradycardia. Dysphasia, visual field defects and facial weakness more common than hemiplegia. Avoid lumbar puncture. Needs surgical drainage. 25% mortality, even if optimally treated.
Encephalitis	May sometimes be confused with stroke. 15% have focal signs. Usually mild preceding febrile illness, headache and drowsiness. Sometimes fits, confusion and gradual-onset coma. Ophthalmoplegia, nystagmus, other cranial nerve, cerebellar and sensory signs possible. Neck may not be stiff. CT scan may be normal. CSF usually abnormal.
Cerebral vasculitis	Difficult to diagnose. Primary or secondary (to temporal arteritis, amphetamines, cocaine, systemic lupus erythematosus, infection, etc.). Results in infarcts or bleeds. Headache prominent, focal neurological deficits, including cranial nerve palsies, or delirium. ESR can be raised, but this and other systemic markers will typically be normal in a primary central nervous system vasculitis. MRI and CSF abnormal. Check autoantibodies. May need angiography or temporal artery/brain/meningeal biopsy. Treat underlying cause and/or high-dose steroids.

Diagnosis	Key features
Venous thrombosis	Difficult to diagnose. Most have headache, half have raised intracranial pressure (nausea, papilloedema), some have focal neurological signs (hemiparesis or paraplegia) or fits. May be secondary to thrombophilia, trauma, infection, or postpartum. CSF is often abnormal (raised pressure, high protein, few red and white cells). CT may show hyperdensity of cortical veins or sinuses, filling defects with contrast (empty delta sign), infarction, disproportionate swelling, and haemorrhage. MR or CT venography is usually diagnostic.
Old stroke, with increased weakness during intercurrent illness	Old neurological signs are often worse during intercurrent illness, especially infections, or appear to be so. Excluding a recurrent stroke is difficult, but rapid return to previous level of function is usual with appropriate treatment. Diffusion-weighted MRI may help.

Features prompting caution include:
- Headache (25% of patients with infarcts have a headache, usually mild)
- Pyrexia
- Malaise or prodromal illness
- Gradual progression over days
- Features of raised intracranial pressure (headache, worst at night, on waking and on coughing, drowsiness, vomiting, hypertension with bradycardia, papilloedema)
- Young age, or absence of vascular risk factors
- Unobtainable or uncertain history.

Some transient neurological conditions can mimic TIA. The most important are:
- *Migraine*. An aura, often a visual disturbance, starts in one homonymous hemi-field, usually develops over about 30 min and lasts less than an hour. Visual phenomena include lights, halos, ziz-zag lines, scotomas, or hemianopias, which build up and may migrate across the entire visual field. Sensory symptoms or hemiparesis can develop with or after visual symptoms, and spread progressively across body parts over several minutes. Dysphasia can occur. Headache, often unilateral and throbbing, typically starts as the aura is resolving, and last 4–72 h, often with nausea and photophobia. Aura may occur without headache, or during the headache, and may last 24 h. Headache may precede the aura. Side may vary with attacks. Basiliar territory symptoms are also possible (dizziness, ataxia, dysarthria).
- *Fits*. Generalized seizures imply loss of consciousness. The patient is rigid and blue during the attack. May be followed by unilateral weakness (Todd's paresis, lasting a few hours to a day or two). Total speech arrest suggests epilepsy, and is unusual in stroke. Partial seizures start in

clear consciousness, but may be secondarily generalized. They may be motor or sensory, with jerking or tingling that tends to build up and spread. Complex partial seizures comprise a disturbance of content of consciousness, with sensory hallucinations (smell or taste, remembered scenes or déjà vu, distorted perceptions of the world), and motor features such as chewing or organized motor activity such as undressing. Dysphasia may occur. Two per cent of patients with stroke have a seizure at onset, half generalized and half partial.

- *Syncopal episodes* have loss of consciousness and postural tone due to a sudden fall in cerebral blood flow. The patient is pale, sweaty, clammy, and floppy, and may jerk. Light-headedness may occur before syncope with dimming or loss of vision. A third have amnesia for the event.
- *Transient global amnesia.* Middle aged or elderly people. Sudden onset. Loss of memory for new information (anterograde amnesia), may also be retrograde amnesia (past events). No loss of personal identity (patients know who they are), problem solving, language, or visuospatial orientation. Look healthy and repetitively ask the same questions. May have headache. Good recovery, recurrence is rare.

Differential diagnosis of coma

- Stroke will sometimes result in sustained unconsciousness (especially when due to bleeding, very large infarcts, or some basilar artery territory strokes). Exclude other causes of coma (metabolic, infective), as some are treatable (Table 1.2).
- Impaired consciousness results from:
  - bilateral cerebral cortical disease (hypoxic, metabolic, toxic, infective, epileptic)
  - impairment of brainstem reticular activating system (lesions of mid-brain to mid-pons, or compression from trans-tentorial herniation due to supra- or infratentorial pressure).
- Large cerebral infarcts with oedema increase intracranial pressure enough to impair cortical function bilaterally, or cause tentorial herniation.
- Evaluation and treatment must be rapid, and must proceed together.
- Look for asymmetry—in tone, movement, and reflexes, and test brainstem function (pupillary responses, doll-eye manoeuvre, corneal and gag reflexes).
- If the pupils are symmetrically reactive, and there are no focal neurological signs, the coma is probably metabolic in origin.
- Coma developing over seconds to minutes suggests a cardiovascular, cerebrovascular, or epileptic cause. If there was recent trauma, consider extradural or subdural haematoma.
- Drug abuse is a cause of otherwise unexplained coma.
- Neurological clues help localization (Table 1.3). But anticholinergic drugs and anoxia can produce large pupils. Opiates and some metabolic diseases can produce (usually reactive) small pupils.
- Anyone in coma needs an urgent CT head scan—unless you are sure of the diagnosis, or that the patient would not have wanted intervention.

Table 1.2 Differential diagnosis of coma

Cause	Clues
Metabolic	
Hypoglycaemia	Glucometer
Diabetic ketoacidosis or hyperosmolar coma	Glucometer, acidosis, ± ketonuria,
Hyper or hyponatraemia	Serum sodium
Hypothermia/hyperthermia	Temperature
Hepatic, uraemic coma	Stigmata, flap, history, blood tests
Septic encephalopathy	Fever, white count, inflammatory markers, focal signs or tests
Myxoedema coma/ thyroid storm	History, clinical state, thyroid function tests
Hypoxia/hypercapnoea	History, pulse oximetry, arterial blood gases
Toxic	
Opiate poisoning	History, constricted pupils, response to naloxone
Benzodiazepines	History, response to flumazenil
Other drug poisoning (alcohol, tricyclics, phenothiazines)	Smell, tachycardia, agitation, hyperreflexia, dilated pupils, blood alcohol.
Drugs of abuse	History, blood or urine toxicology
Carbon monoxide poisoning	Carboxyhaemoglobin (usually >40% to produce coma)
Trauma	
Head injury	History, external signs, CT scan
Shock	
Cardiogenic, pulmonary embolus, hypovolaemic, septic, anaphylactic, drug-induced, Addisonian, neurogenic	Pulse, BP, peripheral perfusion, urine output
Tropical infections	
Malaria, typhoid, rabies, trypanosomiasis	Recent travel, temperature, blood tests
Neurological	
Fits, status epilepticus, postconvulsive	History, convulsions, EEG
Cerebral infarction/ primary intracerebral haemorrhage/SAH	History, signs, CT scan.
Subdural or extradural haematoma	History of trauma. CT scan. Lucid interval after injury.
Meningitis, encephalitis	Fever, malaise, headache, neck and skin signs, CT, lumbar puncture
Hypertensive encephalopathy	BP, fundi, urinalysis, renal function
Brain tumour, abscess	CT scan

Table 1.3 Localizing the cause of coma

Level	Features
Infratentorial	Brainstem causes usually have the most obvious signs and are easiest to diagnose. Look for brainstem signs: Cranial nerve signs ± long tract signs, divergent squint, pupillary and doll's eye reflex loss
Supratentorial (structural lesion)	Asymmetrical long tract signs without brain stem signs (may be false localizing III, IV, or VI if mass effect or aneurysm), focal seizures, conjugate eye deviation.
Toxic-metabolic	Confusion and drowsiness with few motor signs Motor signs symmetrical Pupillary responses preserved Myoclonus, asterixis (flap), tremulousness, and seizures common Acid–base imbalance
Psychogenic	Eyes tight shut Pupils reactive Doll's eye and caloric reflexes preserved Motor tone normal or inconsistent resistance to movement Reflexes normal EEG shows wakefulness

Diagnosing stroke

You need a careful history. If the patient is unconscious, dysphasic, or confused, that is no excuse—ask someone else. If an informant is not immediately present, use the telephone. If there are old hospital case notes available, look at them, and briefly summarize useful information.

You need to know:

- What happened, and what the current symptoms are.
- The time and time-course of onset.
- If it has happened before (previous stroke, TIA).
- Past medical and drug history (prescription, over the counter and illicit—nasal decongestants and cocaine can cause strokes).
- Vascular risk factors.
- Previous functional, occupational, and cognitive ability.
- Information useful for rehabilitation and discharge planning—type of accommodation, cohabitation (and the health of an often-elderly cohabitee), family, and other domestic support.
- Family history of stroke or thrombotic disease (occasionally gives a diagnostic clue, may also reveal previous knowledge, experiences, or expectations).

Some of this can be collected later on, if necessary. But admission is a good opportunity to be thorough.

History taking (and examination) is an inductive process. Use the information you gather to formulate hypotheses about what is going on, which you test with new questions. You want evidence that this is a stroke, and to rule in or rule out other diagnoses. You also want to put the new pathology in context by documenting comorbid conditions, and their disabling consequences.

Examination

General

A thorough general examination is required, because:

- The patient may be very ill, and require securing of the airway, breathing, and circulation before an adequate assessment can be made.
- The possibility of a condition mimicking or causing stroke (atrial fibrillation, malignancy, endocarditis).
- The importance of comorbidity in a generally elderly population.

The cardiovascular system is examined routinely, but the mental state and musculoskeletal systems, in particular, are often overlooked. An admissions ward or Accident and Emergency department is not always the best place to examine these properly.

Initially test cognition using simple orientation (person, place, and time) and short-term memory, or the 10-point abbreviated mental test (AMT, Appendix 1). Later on use the 30-point Folstein MMSE (Appendix 2).

BP may be raised (or very raised), but the ward record over the next hours, days, and weeks will give a better picture of 'usual' BP. The pulse may be slowed in raised intracranial pressure. There may be periodic (Cheyne–Stokes) respiration.

Neurological examination

Is directed at:

- Identifying features that require special precautions (e.g. coma, dysphagia).
- Defining a clinical stroke syndrome (localizing the lesion).
- Quantifying neurological impairments as a baseline for subsequent improvements or deteriorations.
- Raising suspicion of alternative, non-stroke, diagnoses.

The routine examination—cranial nerves, limb tone, power, reflexes, sensation, and cerebellar function should be followed, but some aspects need emphasizing, and others need adapting. You cannot examine co-ordination in a paralysed limb, or assess subtle parietal lobe signs in a drowsy patient.

- At a minimum in an *unconscious, uncomprehending, or uncooperative patient*, and with a little ingenuity, you can record eye movements, facial weakness, limb tone and gross power, and usually reflexes.
- *Level of consciousness*. This is important for prognosis and immediate nursing care. Use the Glasgow Coma Scale (Appendix 3). Describe the response if you cannot remember the numbers. There is a clear problem in underestimating level of consciousness in dysphasia, but it is familiar and well-understood.
- Check for a *stiff neck*, and for evidence of *head trauma*.
- Examine the *fundi* for papilloedema, retinopathy, or subhyaloid haemorrhage.
- If unconscious:
  - check *brainstem function*—pupillary reaction to light, doll's eye movements, corneal reflexes, gag reflex
  - the *caloric reflex* is sometimes useful—can be used after cervical spine trauma

- check the tympanic membrane is intact and there is no wax, then inject 20 ml of ice cold water into the ear canal
- conjugate eye movement towards stimulated ear indicates that the midbrain/pons is intact
- absent or dysconjugate response implies brainstem damage at the level of the pons or sedative drug intoxication
- loss of *pupillary reaction to light* implies a mid-brain lesion. Pontine lesions can cause small but reactive pupils;
- dysconjugate *gaze* indicates a palsy of cranial nerves III, IV, or VI (nuclei in the midbrain and pons) or their connections (medial longitudinal fasciculus), a false localizing sign in raised intracranial pressure, or a mimic such as myasthenia gravis;
- conjugate deviation of the eyes suggests either a frontal lobe infarct on the same side as the direction of gaze, the opposite frontal lobe if an irritative lesion (tumour, haemorrhage), or a pontine lesion in the opposite lateral gaze centre;
- no eye movements at all indicates a pontine lesion (or a mimic such as Guillain–Barré syndrome).
- Check the *visual fields*, upper and lower quadrants. Also, if possible, test for *visual inattention* (sensory extinction—inability to perceive a stimulus when a simultaneous stimulus is presented to the other visual field, in the absence of a visual field defect). Do this with both eyes open, rather than each separately. Wiggling fingers are sufficient for the purpose, rather than coloured pinheads.
- Record *speech* impairment: dysarthria, receptive dysphasia, expressive dysphasia. Test receptive ability (understanding, following commands) first using staged commands with non-verbal response (e.g. 'close your eyes', 'touch your left ear'). If there is reasonable understanding, then test for expressive dysphasia (spontaneous speech, naming).
- Test *swallowing*—with the patient sitting up, give small sips of water, and observe for aspiration. Tap water is more or less sterile. You produce a litre of saliva a day, which must go somewhere, and which is far from sterile. Many hospitals have nurse-delivered swallow testing protocols, which should be used.
- The presence or absence of the gag reflex tells you nothing about the safety of swallowing.
- Examine *motor function*:
  - examine power in the face, arm, and leg;
  - 'pronator drift' is a good test for subtle deficits—the downward drifting and pronation of hands held stretched out horizontally in front, with palms upwards and eyes closed (Fig. 1.1);
  - weakness follows a 'pyramidal distribution'—shoulder abduction, elbow extension, and wrist dorsiflexion will be weaker than corresponding flexor functions, and hip and knee flexion and foot dorsiflexion will be weaker than extensor functions.
- Carefully test the limb *tone* and *reflexes*, especially in mild cases. If the reflexes are very brisk, try the pectoral jerks, and Hoffman's reflex (thumb flexion when the terminal phalanx of the middle finger is flexed under tension then suddenly released with a 'flick'), where asymmetry may be easier to detect (Fig. 1.2).

- Test *co-ordination*, and *gait* if possible. If not, assess head and trunk control.
- Test *sensation*:
  - there may be spinothalamic sensory loss (temperature, pin prick/pain);
  - more useful are some 'cortical sensory modalities', often as part of a search for 'cortical involvement' when identifying a stroke syndrome;
    - stereognosis (identifying objects in the hand)
    - graphaesthesia (identifying numbers traced on the hand)
  - test for sensory inattention (similar to visual inattention, using touch instead of visual stimuli).
- If possible, test for other *cortical or parietal functions*, including:
  - neglect (Albert's test—line cancellation, drawing a clock face, or double-headed daisy);
  - apraxia (drawing tasks—intersecting pentagons, five-pointed star);
  - sometimes specific dyscalculia (sums), dyslexia (reading), or dysgraphia (writing);
  - body image and proprioception can be assessed using the 'thumb-finding test' (affected arm supported in front, eyes closed, the patient is asked to find his thumb with his unaffected hand).

Some of these tests can wait for a few days. However, signs may resolve rapidly.

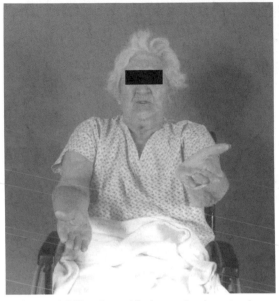

Fig. 1.1 Pronator drift. The right arm drifts downwards and pronates when held out in front with eyes shut.

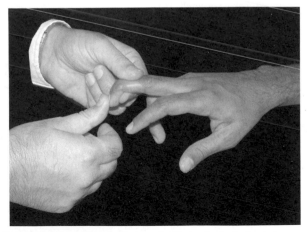

Fig. 1.2 Hoffman's reflex. After flexing and suddenly releasing the terminal phalanx, the thumb flexes if the reflex is positive.

Investigations

- First check blood glucose with a portable glucometer (e.g. BM stick).
- Get a CT head scan (or MRI) as soon as possible after admission, unless the diagnosis is certain and the patient is moribund. The scan is to diagnose or exclude bleeds and stroke-mimics rather than to confirm infarction.
- The CT scan should be urgent if thrombolysis is possible, or if there is suspicion of:
  - trauma
  - cerebellar haematoma
  - SAH
  - raised intracranial pressure
  - if level of consciousness is deteriorating
  - there is undiagnosed coma
  - if the patient is on anticoagulants, or needs anticoagulation (or antithrombotics, if a bleed is suspected).
- Blood count, electrolytes, including calcium, glucose, renal, liver, and thyroid function, ESR or C-reactive protein and urinalysis should be done routinely. Check coagulation if on anticoagulants, or if proposing them, and cholesterol if within 2 days of the stroke.
- Electrocardiogram in everyone.
- Ideally get an echocardiogram in potentially embolic (partial anterior and posterior circulation) strokes. However, the call for echocardiography is high, and local services may limit this to cases where there is other clinical or ECG evidence of heart disease.
- You are unlikely to get a technically decent chest X-ray. In any case you are more likely to diagnose malignancy from the CT head scan than the chest X-ray. Don't request routinely unless there are specific chest problems or signs you want to investigate (e.g. unexplained fever or presumed aspiration pneumonia).
- Carotid duplex scan if anterior circulation stroke resulting in no more than minor disability, and the patient would be willing to undergo carotid endarterectomy. May also detect carotid dissection.
- Contrast, CT or MR angiography—to diagnose dissection, as a prelude to carotid endarterectomy, or to investigate intracranial bleeding (from an aneurysm or arteriovenous malformation) when neurosurgery is contemplated.
- Ambulatory ECG (24-h tape) is rarely necessary. Some evidence suggests that paroxysmal atrial fibrillation can be detected in association with stroke on 24-h ECG monitoring that will not be detected otherwise, but the diagnostic yield is poor. Consider it where the aetiology remains unclear, and cardiac embolism is suspected (multiple cortical lesions).
- Additional tests may be required in younger stroke patients (<50 years). See section 'Stroke in younger adults', p. 24.

Clinical subtypes

Stroke is a mixed bag of pathologies. These include intracerebral and sub-arachnoid bleeding, and infarction. Infarction divides between large vessel disease, small end-artery (lacunar) disease, cardioembolism and rare causes such as venous infarction, vasculitis, and infective endocarditis.

Primary intracerebral haemorrhage (Table 1.4)

Acute bleeds have some characteristic features:
- apoplectic onset (sudden loss of consciousness)
- headache
- vomiting
- stiff neck

Unfortunately, these, and various scoring systems derived from combinations of them (such as the Guy's diagnostic and Siriraj scores) are insufficiently accurate for clinical use. Small bleeds can be clinically indistinguishable from infarcts.

An early CT scan is required to make the diagnosis. The request should be urgent where SAH is suspected (to initiate medical management, and part of the work-up to exclude meningitis). Haematomas absorb over 10–30 days. Leave the scan longer than a week, and a small bleed may have resolved on CT, although MRI can still detect haemoglobin break-down products for many months.

Infarcts

Pathological mechanisms

A good level of diagnostic acumen and clinical suspicion is needed to detect rare but treatable causes of infarction such as infective endocarditis (peripheral stigmata, new murmurs, raised inflammatory markers, positive blood cultures), cerebral vasculitis, thrombophilia, or venous infarction.

Once these have been excluded, we are left with the majority of patients, who have cerebral infarction due to arterial thrombosis or embolism.

If we are to direct further investigation and management logically, ideally we need to know more than just that a stroke has occurred. Table 1.5 gives some different pathological mechanisms. In practice, 20–40% of causes remain undetermined despite comprehensive work-up. Sometimes, however, we can work out exactly why the stroke occurred.

Oxfordshire Community Stroke Project (OCSP) (Bamford) Classification (Table 1.6)

The OCSP or Bamford anatomical classification localizes stroke lesions on clinical grounds, and indicates likely pathology and prognosis.
- POCIs are mostly thrombotic (80%), the rest embolic (20%).
- LACI are due to thrombotic occlusions of small, deep, end-arteries.
- PACI are predominantly embolic.
- TACI split between embolic (two-thirds) and *in-situ* thrombosis (one-third).

Clinical stroke type agrees well with anatomical localization on CT scan (although lacunar and partial anterior circulation strokes are least reliably distinguished).

Table 1.4 Pathology of intracerebral haemorrhage

Type	Features
Charcot–Bouchard microaneurysms	Lipohyalinosis, often associated with hypertension, causes weakness of the walls of small perforating arteries, usually to the basal ganglia, thalamus, or pons
Amyloid angiopathy	Commonest cause of lobar haemorrhage in the over 60's. Affects small arteries particularly in the meninges and superficial cortex. Arteries are weakened by fibrinoid degeneration, amyloid deposition, segmental dilatation, and micro-aneurysm formation. Affects men and women equally, especially those with dementia. Resulting haematoma is usually superficial and lobar. Often recur.
Berry aneurysms	Comprise majority of intracranial aneurysms. Thin-walled saccular dilatation of the arteries, may be multiloculated if large. Probably acquired rather than congenital. Most are small. Found in 2–5% of autopsies. Associated with age, hypertension, and atheroma. Found at distal end of the arteries, mainly at circle of Willis—carotid tree 75%; basilar tree 10%; both 15%. Rupture causes SAH, but may extend into the brain substance or ventricles.
Fusiform aneurysms	Found on atheromatous large arteries (internal carotid, basilar) in elderly people, due to replacement of the muscular layer by fibrous tissue. A common site is the supraclinoid segment of the internal carotid artery. A complication is compression of structures in the cavernous sinus wall.
Arteriovenous malformations	Consist of a mass of enlarged and tortuous vessels. Supplied by one or more large arteries. Drained by one or more large veins. They are congenital and may run in families. Present with recurrent headaches, epilepsy, SAH or intracerebral haemorrhages. Commonest site is on the middle cerebral artery.
Secondary haemorrhage	Due to anticoagulant therapy, thrombolytic therapy (e.g. for heart attack), haemorrhagic disease, bleeding into tumours or mycotic aneurysms, or haemorrhagic transformation of an infarct

Table 1.5 Pathology of cerebral infarction

Type	Features
Cardiac emboli	About 20% of ischaemic strokes. Causes include valvular disease (mitral stenosis and prosthetic valves), atrial fibrillation, mural thrombus after myocardial infarction, left ventricular aneurysm, dilated cardiomyopathy, atrial myxoma, patent foramen ovale with paradoxical embolism of venous thrombi. Typically results in a peripherally located, wedge-shaped infarcts, often becoming haemorrhagic. Can involve multiple arterial distributions.
Large vessel disease	Atherosclerosis of aorta, common carotid and internal carotid artery. Stenosis, plaque rupture and ulceration, platelet aggregation, and red cell thrombus formation, may cause occlusion or provide a source of emboli. Internal carotid artery clot may propagate into the middle cerebral artery. Otherwise perfusion is dependent on collaterals from the circle of Willis.
Small vessel (lacunar) disease	Lipohyalinosis or micro-atheroma of small end-arteries, associated with hypertension, diabetes mellitus, or hyperlipidaemia.
Arterial dissection (carotid or vertebral)	About 5% of ischaemic stroke under 65 years of age, sometimes following trauma or unusual neck movements. May have pain in the neck or face, and an ipsilateral Horner's syndrome.
Arterial boundary-zone (watershed) infarction	May complicate hypotension or cardiac arrest. Damage is variable. Usually bilateral, often parieto-occipital (between middle cerebral artery and posterior cerebral artery territories), causing cortical blindness, visual disorientation, amnesia, agnosia. The anterior cerebral artery/middle cerebral artery boundary can be compromised due to unilateral internal carotid artery stenosis or occlusion, causing predominant leg weakness or sensory loss, with facial sparing. Other patterns are possible, including cortical sensory loss, dysphasia, hemianopia, motor weakness.
Post-SAH	Infarction occurs within 4–12 days in 25% of patients with SAH, due to arterial spasm
Rare causes	Infective endocarditis, vasculitis (e.g. giant cell arteritis, systemic lupus erythematosus), subclavian steal, hyperviscosity and prothrombotic conditions, postpartum, iatrogenic causes (internal jugular cannulation, cerebral angiography or cardiac catheterization)

Table 1.6 Oxfordshire Community Stroke Project Stroke Classification

Type	Features
POCI	Cranial nerve deficit with contralateral hemiparesis or sensory deficit, or bilateral stroke, or disorders of conjugate eye movement, or isolated cerebellar stroke, or isolated homonymous hemianopia
LACI	Pure motor or pure sensory deficit affecting two of three of face, arm, and leg, or sensorimotor stroke (basal ganglia and internal capsule), or ataxic hemiparesis (cerebellar-type ataxia with ipsilateral pyramidal signs—internal capsule or pons); or dysarthria plus clumsy hand, or acute onset movement disorders (hemi-chorea, hemiballismus—basal ganglia)
TACI	1. New higher cerebral function dysfunction: dysphasia/dyscalculia/apraxia/neglect/visuospatial problems plus 2. Homonymous visual field defect, plus 3. Ipsilateral motor and/or sensory deficit of at least two areas of face, arm and leg. In the presence of impaired consciousness, higher cerebral function and visual fields deficits are assumed.
PACI	Two of the three components of TACI, or isolated dysphasia or other cortical dysfunction, or motor/sensory loss more limited than for a LACI

Lancet 1991; **337**: 1521–6.

Brainstem strokes

Brainstem strokes can be missed, but are also overdiagnosed, because the individual elements are non-specific (like diplopia or vertigo), meaning that they can be caused by a number of different pathologies. It is the specific combination of neurological signs and symptoms that indicate the focal nature of the lesion. Some of these patterns are given in Table 1.7.

Basilar artery occlusion

Complete occlusion has a mortality of 80%, but partial occlusion is also possible. The clinical course is stuttering and progressive, over days to weeks. Causes can be *in situ* thrombosis, embolism, and vertebral artery dissection.

Symptoms and signs are variable, depending on the level of the occlusion (i.e. any of the posterior circulation strokes), and the state of collateral flow. Symptoms include:

- vertigo
- headache
- oculomotor and limb weakness
- drowsiness or coma
- dysarthria.

Up to 70% have hemiparesis or quadriparesis; 40% have pupillary abnormalities, oculomotor signs (III, VI, internuclear ophthalmoplegia, conjugate gaze defects), and pseudobulbar palsy (facial weakness, dysphonia, dysarthria, dysphagia).

'Top of the basilar syndrome' is usually due to an embolus. Presents with abnormal conscious level, visual symptoms (hallucinations, cortical blindness), abnormal eye movements (usually of vertical gaze), third nerve palsy and pupillary abnormalities, and abnormal motor movements or posturing.

Coma with oculomotor abnormalities and quadriplegia indicates pontine damage due to mid-basilar occlusion.

'Locked-in' syndrome comprises complete paralysis apart from blinking and vertical eye movements. The patient is aware and alert (i.e. can potentially respond purposefully to external stimuli). Caused by proximal basilar occlusion.

MRI and MRA are the investigations of choice.

Table 1.7 Brainstem strokes

Level		Neurological signs by side		Eponym
		Ipsilateral	Contralateral	
Mid-brain	Dorsolateral	Horner's ± cerebellar	Total sensory loss	
	Paramedian	III	Cerebellar ataxia, hemichorea	Benedikt
	Basal	III	Hemiplegia	Weber
Pons	Dorsolateral	Horner's, cerebellar, ±VII, ±V (sensory), ± gaze palsy	Spinothalamic sensory loss	
	Paramedian	VI, gaze palsy	± spinothalamic sensory loss	
	Basal	VI, LMN VII, hemiplegia	± UMN VII	Millard–Gubler
	Bilateral ventral	Locked-in syndrome		
Medulla	Lateral	Horner's, facial spinothalamic loss (pain, temperature), cerebellar ataxia, LMN VII, VIII (vertigo, vomiting), IX, X, (dysphagia)	Corporal spinothalamic loss	Wallenberg
	Central	XII	Hemiplegia, dorsal column sensory loss	

LMN, lower motor neuron; UMN, upper motor neuron.

Stroke in younger adults

Ten per cent of strokes occur in people under 50 years of age.

Be on the alert for something unusual (Table 1.8). There is little fundamentally different about stroke in younger people. You still need to arrive at an explanation for what has happened, and many of the rarer causes of stroke also arise in older adults. About 30% of strokes in younger adults remain unexplained despite investigation.

Atherosclerotic vascular disease does occur in adults under 50, but is relatively less common. Bleeds, cardiogenic stroke, and stroke-mimics are all proportionately more common.

Particular additional diagnoses to consider are:
- arterial dissection
- substance abuse
- bleeding disorders and prothrombotic states
- vasculitis.

Table 1.8 Additional tests in younger patients

Condition	Test	Comments
Arterial dissection	Neck MRI, MRA, angiography, duplex scan	High index of suspicion in patients under 50, otherwise look out for clinical clues
Substance abuse	History, blood and urine toxicology	Cocaine, amphetamine, and heroin. Cause vasospasm, hypertension, or vasculitis. Watch for endocarditis
Sickle cell disease	Haemoglobin electrophoresis	Afro-Caribbean people
Thrombophilia	Protein S and C deficiencies, antithrombin III, factor V Leiden/PC resistance, prothrombin 20210A	Usually cause venous thromboses, but sometimes arterial disease, or cause paradoxical embolism
Antiphospholipid syndrome	Persistent (over 6 weeks) anticardiolipin antibody, or lupus anticoagulant, with thrombosis, fetal loss, thrombocytopenia	May be primary or secondary (connective tissue disorders, infections, drugs). Mostly venous thromboses, sometimes arterial. 20% of thromboses are cerebral (arterial or venous). Recurrence common (9% per year)
Hyperhomo-cysteinaemia	Homocysteine (random or post-methionine load)	Treat with folic acid and pyridoxine
Oestrogens	History (postpartum, combined oral contraceptive, HRT)	May cause venous sinus thrombosis

Table 1.8 continued

Waldenström's macroglobulinaemia	ESR, protein electrophoresis, plasma viscosity	More often hyperviscosity syndrome (drowsy, headache, ataxia, diplopia, visual blurring, dysarthria)
Malignancy	History, blood tests, imaging	Especially gastrointestinal, breast and gynaecological. Warfarin may not control
Bleeding disorders	FBC, prothrombin time/ INR, APTT, fibrin degradation products	Anticoagulants, thrombolytics, leukaemia, platelet disorders, disseminated intravascular coagulation, haemophilia
Vasculitis	Clinical features (headache, weight loss, fever, malaise, jaw claudication, scalp tenderness, polymyalgia, rash, joint or renal problems, anaemia); ESR; double-stranded-DNA; anti-neutrophil cytoplasmic antibody; temporal artery, skin, renal, or brain biopsy; MRI	Can be primary, otherwise connective tissue disorders, Sjögren's, Behçet's, sarcoid. Diagnosis may be known. MRI shows meningeal inflammation and areas of patchy infarction or haemorrhage. Angiography may be helpful but is non-specific.
Patent foramen ovale with paradoxical embolism	Bubble contrast echocardiography with Valsalva manoeuvre	Lower threshold for transoesophageal echo if no likely non-cardiac source, but difficult to establish causality
Cerebral autosomal dominant arteriopathy with subcortical infarcts and leucoencephalopathy	MRI	Hereditary small vessel arteriopathy. Presents in middle age. Migraine, recurrent lacunar strokes, and later dementia
Mitochondrial encephalomyopathy with lactic acidosis and stroke-like episodes (MELAS)	MRI, plasma and CSF lactate, genetics	Typically produces strokes in non-arterial distributions. Often occipital lobe strokes at very young age (children), fits, multiple other problems

Carotid and vertebral arterial dissection

The arterial wall splits, blood enters the media, resulting in an intramural haematoma, and a true and a false lumen. Ischaemic stroke results from:
- occlusion of the true lumen by the dissection or thrombus, or
- embolism from thrombus within the true lumen.

Spontaneous arterial dissection occurs in atheroma, cystic medial necrosis, fibromuscular dysplasia, Ehlers–Danlos and Marfan's syndromes. Intracranial (vertebrobasilar) dissection can cause SAH.

Features include:
- History of neck trauma (including rotation, hyperextension, and penetrating injuries), but this is absent from most.
- Pain may be present in one of the following areas:
  - face
  - around the eye
  - neck (ipsilateral to carotid dissection)
  - unusual unilateral headache
  - occiput and back of the neck (vertebral dissection)
- May have no neurological signs.
- 10–20% experience TIA.
- Ipsilateral Horner's syndrome due to damage to the sympathetic fibres around the internal carotid artery (50%, Fig 1.3a).
- Unilateral lower cranial nerve palsies (12%, particularly hypoglossal, due to pressure from the internal carotid wall at the base of the skull).
- Contralateral motor, visual or higher cortical function deficits.
- Note that the combination of ipsilateral cranial nerve and contralateral pyramidal lesions mimics brainstem strokes.
- The pain and Horner's syndrome may precede stroke by a few days to 4 weeks.

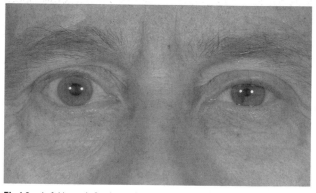

Fig 1.3a: Left Horner's Syndrome (partial ptosis, small pupil) in a right-handed man with a left unilateral headache and aphasia.

- Consider skin and joint hyperextensibility, abnormal scars, and retinal abnormalities.
- The definitive investigation is cerebral angiography, MRA, or CTA, but may also be seen on carotid duplex scanning and neck MRI (Fig. 1.3b–e).
- If the carotid is completely occluded by the dissection, imaging is non-specific.
- Imaging must be done within days of symptom onset, because the dissection often resolves spontaneously.
- Recurs at about 1% per year.

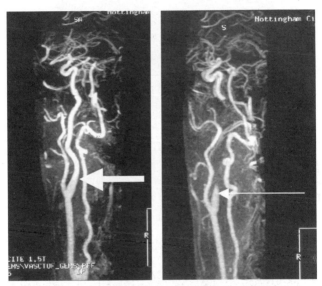

Fig 1.3b and c: MR angiograms demonstrate a normal right internal carotid artery (thick arrow) and an occluded left internal carotid artery (thin arrow).

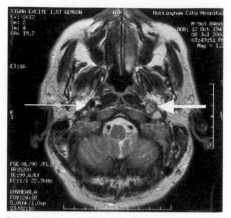

Fig 1.3d: T-2 weighted brain MRI. The left internal carotid artery has a small, dark, central residual lumen containing white thrombus. The surrounding white ring is intramural thrombus ('crescent sign', thick arrow). Compare with the normal flow-void (dark) of the right internal carotid artery (thin arrow)

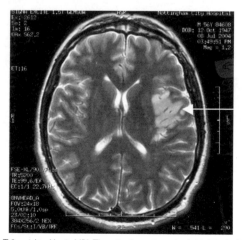

Fig 1.3e: T-2 weighted brain MRI. There is a hyper-intensity (white) in the leftt insular cortex and pars opercularis, indicating infarction at the site of the language centre (arrow)

Summary

1. Stroke is a clinical syndrome—a rapidly developing episode of focal or global neurological dysfunction, lasting longer than 24 h or leading to death, and of presumed vascular origin.
2. Diagnosis can be difficult. The deficit may progress over 24 h or more, the presentation may be atypical, and some alternative diagnoses are difficult to make.
3. At least 10% of presumed strokes reaching hospital will have another diagnosis.
4. The neurological deficits depend on where the stroke is and how big it is. Hence, it is quite variable, but a number of distinct patterns can be identified.
5. The OCSP clinical classification gives useful information about the extent of neurological deficit, aetiology, prognosis, and recurrence rates.
6. An attempt should be made at elucidating the pathology underlying the stroke—unless the patient is clearly moribund and no active intervention is contemplated. Most important are the clinical stroke subtype, CT or MRI scans, blood glucose, electrolytes, ECG and inflammatory markers.
7. If there is pain or neck trauma, or in younger patients, consider arterial dissection. In younger patients also consider the possibility of substance abuse.

Chapter 2

What to do in the first few days

How health services help

Health care has seven main functions (Table 2.1). Tasks are shared between doctors, nurses, and other health professionals.

The first day

The first task on seeing any patient is to make a rapid evaluation of immediate resuscitation needs, and act if necessary. Assess:
- airway
- breathing
- circulation.

Make sure that the patient is free from immediate physical danger (falling off the trolley or out of bed?), and undue distress. After that, tasks for the first day include:
- Making, or confirming, the diagnosis.
- Documenting comorbid conditions or complications.
- Understanding the immediate context of the disease, including its severity and resulting disabilities, other complicating medical factors, and sufficient background social information to allow decisions on the need for admission to hospital, or the scope for early discharge.
- Ordering initial investigations.
- Making risk assessments for pressure areas, moving and handling, nutrition, bed rails, and falls.
- Instigating plans for maintaining oxygenation, relief of pressure areas, feeding and hydration, bladder and bowel management, and venous thrombosis prevention.
- Monitoring.
- Initial specific medical management.
- Management of immediate complications and comorbid conditions.
- Making initial referrals to rehabilitation therapists.
- Communicating the diagnosis and plans to patients, their relatives, medical and nursing colleagues.

Prewritten care pathways can help ensure that assessments and interventions are systematic, comprehensive, and made at the right time (Appendix 4).

Table 2.1 Seven functions of health care

Function	Examples in stroke care
Prevention of disease, or complications of disease	Manipulation of vascular risk factors; aspirin or anticoagulants in vascular disease; prevention of pressure sores, dehydration, malnutrition, aspiration pneumonia, venous thrombosis, joint contractures, institutionalization
Cure of disease, or complications of disease	Thrombolysis in acute stroke; antibiotics for infections; healing of pressure sores; feeding in malnutrition; antidepressants for biological depression (?)
Prolonging life, deferring death	Organized multidisciplinary stroke care; antibiotics for pneumonia; aspirin and antihypertensive drugs as secondary prevention
Palliation of unpleasant symptoms	Analgesic for pain; mouth care if nil by mouth; management of anxiety and depression; drugs for spasticity; management of incontinence; many treatments of comorbid conditions
Maximize physical and social function (rehabilitation)	Physiotherapy, OT, rehabilitation nursing, speech therapy, goal setting, discharge planning, environmental changes
Information	Explanation of diagnosis and its effects; advising on secondary prevention; giving prognosis
Support for families and other carers	Reassurance; concern, empathy, and sympathy; positive outlook; realistic planning; training in care-giving

Whether and where to admit?

The great majority of stroke patients should be admitted to hospital. Do so unless:

- Functional impairment is minimal.
- The patient can be seen in an appropriate clinic within a week. The clinic should be able to confirm the diagnosis, identify residual disabilities and secondary prevention needs. Such clinics should have immediate access to CT head and carotid duplex scanning.
- The patient has pre-existing severe chronic disabilities, often a nursing homes resident. Admission may have little to offer in terms of nursing care, sensible investigation, or treatment. In experienced hands this can represent good, humane, and appropriate care. Such a decision is not easy to make, and may require specialist consultation to support it. If handled poorly, decisions not to admit can be discriminatory, or lead to self-fulfilling prophesies (outcome is poor not because it was inevitable, but because potentially useful treatments were not given).

Ideally admission should be directly to a specialist acute stroke unit. Otherwise try to transfer to an acute stroke unit within 24 h.

The rationale for hospital admission is:

- Patients value admission. They and their families are suddenly met with frightening or bewildering symptoms (such as hemiparesis and dysphasia), need reassurance that they are being cared for, and have the support of people who have seen it before, know what they are doing, and can facilitate return to normal abilities.
- Co-ordinated, specialist, in-patient stroke care prevents unnecessary deaths, disability, and dependency (compared with care on general medical wards), suggesting that some aspects of hospital care are important in determining outcomes.
- A controlled trial in the 1980s found that a home-based care team increased admission rates, probably by uncovering previously unmet needs.
- A recent randomized trial compared admission to a stroke ward, home-based, multidisciplinary specialist care, and a peripatetic team who supported management on general medical wards. It found decisively in favour of the stroke ward (Box 2.1).

Box 2.1 Orpington models of care trial

- 467 acute patients within 72 h of stroke, with persisting disability, but who were fit enough to consider home management, were randomized between stroke unit care, specialist home care supported by a stroke physician, or general ward care supported by a mobile stroke team.
- 34% of the domiciliary group were subsequently admitted to the hospital stroke unit.
- Mortality or institutionalization at 1 year were 14% for the stroke unit, 24% for home care (including those transferred to the stroke unit) and 30% for supported general ward care. The main reduction was in mortality.
- Proportions alive without severe disability at 1 year were 85% (in-patient stroke unit), 71% (specialized home care) and 66% (general medical ward with mobile stroke team).

Lancet 2000; **356**: 894–9

Management of coma

- You may admit patients who are unconscious, with a working diagnosis of stroke. Initially the diagnosis is uncertain.
- If the diagnosis is stroke, the outlook is poor but not hopeless. Toxic, metabolic, or other comorbidity may be complicating the picture.
- The aim is to provide resuscitation and supportive treatment while a diagnosis is made, and allowing definitive management to be instituted.
- If maintaining the airway is at risk consult an anaesthetist or intensivist urgently, unless you are sure of the diagnosis, and that active intervention is inappropriate.

Initial management of coma

- Assessment and diagnosis must proceed at the same time as resuscitation.
- Secure the airway (recovery position, oral airway). Intubate if need be:
  - respiration may deteriorate suddenly;
  - intubation protects the airway against aspirating vomit;
  - perform a rapid neurological examination first if sedation is required.
- Give oxygen 28% by mask or nasal cannulae.
- Monitor pulse, BP, and respiration rate and pattern, pulse oximetry, and/or arterial blood gases. Act to correct if need be, aiming to keep oxygen saturation >95%.
- Check blood glucose. If low (<3 mmol/l), give 50 ml 50% glucose IV (plus B vitamins/'Pabrinex'® IV if alcoholic or malnourished).
- Terminate seizures with IV lorazepam (2 mg repeated twice if necessary) or IV diazepam (10 mg, repeated twice if necessary). If seizures persist, or for maintenance, use IV phenytoin (loading dose 15 mg/kg at <50 mg/min with ECG monitoring, then 100 mg tds).
- Rapid neurological examination:
  - hand drop over head (to exclude malingering);
  - neck stiffness (unless cervical spine trauma possible);
  - pupil size and reactivity to light;
  - eye movement assessment (doll's eyes manoeuvre);
  - response to painful stimulus (knuckle to sternum, nail bed pressure);
  - limb tone, movement and plantar responses.
- Take blood for blood count, culture, biochemistry, including calcium, renal, thyroid and liver function, and lactate.
- Start IV normal saline (1 litre over 8 h, unless clinically hypovolaemic, or in overt heart failure).
- Insert a urinary catheter only if you need urine for toxicology screening, or to measure urine output.
- Treat hyperthermia (tepid sponge) or hypothermia (space blanket).
- If overdose is suspected, empty stomach (if within 6–12 h depending on likely drug involved). Intubate first, then use gastric lavage and activated charcoal 50–100 g.
- Arrange urgent CT head.
- Monitor conscious level using the Glasgow Coma Scale.

Presumed supratentorial mass lesions with raised intracranial pressure

- Intubate and hyperventilate to lower intracranial pressure in the short term (30 min to a few hours, by vasoconstricting and reducing intracerebral blood volume).
- Tilt head up (30°).
- Give 20% mannitol 0.5–1 g/kg (about 250 ml), over 15 min (reduces intracranial pressure in 20–60 min and lasts 4–6 h). Usually a short-term measure while a diagnosis is made. Monitor blood electrolytes.
- If stroke is the cause, hyperventilation and mannitol are not particularly effective.
- Give dexamethasone 4 mg IV (6 hourly) if CT head shows vasogenic oedema secondary to tumour or abscess. Effective in several hours. Ineffective in stroke.
- Refer to a neurosurgeon if a tumour or abscess is suspected, and consider referral if there is a haematoma.

Infratentorial lesions

- Reduce intracranial pressure as above.
- Refer to neurosurgeon for decompression of cerebellar haematoma, or cerebellar infarct with oedema.
- Treat intrinsic brainstem tumours with dexamethasone in the first instance.

Toxic or metabolic coma

- Exclude/treat hypoglycaemia.
- Severe metabolic acidosis (pH <7.0) give IV sodium bicarbonate 1 mEq/kg (1.26% is 150 mEq/l and can be given peripherally).
- If carbon monoxide poisoning give 100% oxygen (consider transfer to hyperbaric oxygen facility).
- If CT normal, consider a lumbar puncture.
- If history, signs, or CSF suggest acute bacterial meningitis, treat according to microbiological advice.
- Drug overdose—mainly supportive, but specific antidotes may help:
  - Contact the specialist regional toxicology centre for advice.
  - Opiates—naloxone IV 400 μg repeated at 2-min intervals up to maximum 10 mg. Short duration of action, and may need repeating or infusing.
  - Benzodiazepines—flumazenil 200 μg IV, then 100 μg at 60-s intervals, if required, maximum dose 1 mg. Short acting and may need repeating or infusing (100–400 μg/h). Response can be dramatic, but avoid if also taken tricyclic antidepressants (risk of seizures).

Acute medical management of cerebral infarcts

Strategies include:
- Diagnostic accuracy and aetiological understanding.
- Reperfusion (thrombolysis).
- Physiological normalization (controlling BP, maintaining oxygenation, normalizing blood glucose, reducing pyrexia, fluid rehydration).
- Prevention, or early detection and treatment, of neurological and medical complications.

Diagnosis should be reviewed by a senior clinician with expertise in stroke within 24 h of admission, and sooner if necessary.

Most recommendations are likely to be of benefit on a balance of probabilities rather than proven beyond doubt in randomized trials.

Thrombolysis

Thrombolysis can reduce death and disability, but only if given to highly selected patients who can reach hospital, be assessed, have a CT scan, and have treatment started within 3 h (Boxes 2.2 and 2.3):
- Thrombolysis with IV recombinant tissue plasminogen activator (tPA or alteplase; 0.9 mg/kg, maximum 90 mg, 10% as bolus, rest over 1 h) in the absence of contraindications.
- The risk is doing more harm than good. Symptomatic intracranial haemorrhages occur in 6% after thrombolysis compared with 1% with placebo. The hospital must have the staffing and infrastructure to deliver thrombolysis safely to an agreed protocol. There is a long list of contraindications and cautions, and monitoring must be rigorous. For centres giving thrombolysis, target 'door-to-needle time' is less than 1 h.
- Intra-arterial thrombolysis for proximal middle cerebral artery occlusion within 6 h of onset with pro-urokinase is similarly effective where available (interventional neuroradiologists).
- Appendices 5–7 give details of medical work-up, a suitability checklist, and monitoring requirements.

Other acute medical management

Guidelines for immediate medical treatment and management of specific neurological complications are given in Table 2.2.

Cerebral autoregulation is lost in areas of evolving infarction, so blood flow is passively dependent on mean arterial pressure. The first objective after stroke is to avoid drops in BP. An arbitrary upper limit of 220–240/120–130 mmHg is set (overperfusion promotes cerebral oedema), with the proviso that BP reduction should be slow and not go below target (180/105).

Observational evidence suggests best outcomes are with initial systolic pressures of 140–180 mmHg, which corresponds with recommendations based on cerebral blood flow.

Existing antihypertensive medication can be continued, but should be stopped if BP is below target.

Box 2.2 Trials of tPA (alteplase) in acute stroke

- The National Institute of Neurological Disorders and Stroke (NINDS) trial randomized 624 patients to 0.9 mg/kg tPA or placebo, half within 90 min of stroke and half within 180 min.
- There was a small benefit with thrombolysis on a 42-point neurological score, the NIH Stroke Scale (median scores 8 vs. 12), and a small reduction in mortality in the tPA group (17% vs. 21%, $P = 0.30$).
- More patients had complete or almost complete recovery on four outcome scales, including the Rankin scale (43% vs. 27%). Thirteen to 16% experienced a more favourable 3-month outcome with tPA compared with placebo. The number needed to treat per favourable outcome was six to nine patients.
- The European Co-operative Acute Stroke Study (ECASS-1) randomized 620 patients to 1.1 mg/kg tPA or placebo, within 6 h of stroke onset. There was a small benefit for tPA in neurological and functional outcomes, at the cost of an increased mortality rate. Thirty-day mortality was 18% vs. 13%, but 36% of the tPA group were independent on the Rankin score vs. 29% for placebo (odds ratio 1.2, 95% CI 0.98–1.35).
- ECASS-2 randomized 800 patients to 0.9 mg/kg tPA or placebo within 6 h of stroke onset. Strokes were less severe than those in ECASS-1. 10.6% of patients died within 90 days in each group. There was a small advantage for tPA in terms of independent Rankin scores (40% vs. 37% for Rankin scores 0–1, or 54% vs. 46% for Rankin scores 0–2).
- Data from 2775 patients randomized in these trials [plus the ATLANTIS (Alteplase Thrombolysis for Acute Noninterventional Therapy in Ischemic Stroke) trials] have been pooled and re-analysed. The outcome was full, or nearly full, recovery defined by the Rankin (0–1), NIHSS (0–1), or Barthel (>95/100) scores after 3 months. Benefit from treatment decreased with time from stroke onset. For treatment within 0–90 min, odds ratio for favourable outcomes was 2.8 (95% CI 1.8–4.5), for 91–180 min 1.6 (1.1–2.2), for 181–270 min 1.4 (0.1–1.9), and for 271–360 min 1.2 (0.9–1.5). Chances of very poor outcomes (death or severe dependency) increased slightly with onset to treatment time.
- Another overview estimated an RR for death or dependency of 0.66 (95% CI 0.53–0.83) for patients treated within 3 h, absolute risk reduction 50% vs. 60% (95% CI for difference 5–16%). Six per cent of thrombolysed patients experienced intracerebral bleeds, half fatal, compared to 1% for placebo.

Lancet 2004; **363**: 768–74

Box 2.3 Healthcare system requirements for delivering thrombolysis

- *Public knowledge*: acute onset of focal neurological signs prompts emergency attendance at hospital or calling an ambulance.
- *General practitioners*: direct acute focal neurology to hospital immediately.
- *Ambulance service*: priority attendance at calls and transfer to hospital, oxygenation, IV hydration, blood sugar check, question witnesses for time of onset, advance warning of arrival to hospital Emergency Department staff.
- *Hospital emergency department*: initiate assessment, alert dedicated stroke team, order emergency CT scan, IV access.
- *CT scanner and reporting*: 24-h immediate access. Follow-up CT scan availability for complications. Immediate reliable reporting of scans by radiologist or stroke physician/ neurologist.
- *On-call stroke or neurological team*:
  - full work-up (Appendix 5), blood tests;
  - medical stabilization;
  - head scan interpretation;
  - complete suitability checklist (Appendix 6);
  - consent (or assessment of best interests);
  - immediate access to tPA.
- *Ward*: Monitoring facilities and trained staff (Appendix 7).
- *Governance*: Monitoring and audit of indications, process, complications, and outcomes.

Table 2.2 Acute treatment for physiological normalization

Abnormality	Intervention
Fluid balance	IV saline or Ringer's infusion, central venous pressure 8–10 cm H_2O. Less if raised intracranial pressure.
Low BP (<140/90)	Control arrhythmias. Stop antihypertensive drugs. IV fluids to maintain filling pressure, target BP 160–180/90–100.
Sustained high BP >230/120, after 1st hour	Reduce slowly to 180/105 with oral ACE inhibitor. IV labetolol in 10 mg doses up to 150 mg, or IV nitrates (isosorbide dinitrate 1–10 mg/h). Avoid subingual nifedipine.
Mild-moderate hypoxia	2–4 l/min oxygen by mask or nasal cannulae, keep SaO_2 >95%
Severe hypoxia, unconscious	Intubation and ventilation (taking account of prognosis, comorbidity, and patient's wishes)
Glucose >10 mmol/l	IV insulin sliding scale, reduce to <10 mmol/l
Pyrexia >37.5°C	Paracetamol 1 g po/pr qds, antibiotics if evidence of infection
Comorbid conditions	Optimize
Raised intracranial pressure	Mild dehydration, head up 30°, 10% glycerol or mannitol, consider decompressive craniotomy for extensive middle cerebral artery or cerebellar infarction

SaO_2, oxygen saturation. European Stroke Initiative, http://www.eusi-stroke.com/recommenations/rc_overview.shtml

BP should not be reduced in the first hour, unless there is:
- Hypertensive encephalopathy (very high BP, drowsiness and confusion, retinopathy and papilloedema).
- Hypertensive heart failure or acute MI.
- Acute renal failure.
- Aortic dissection.

Aspirin

Aspirin, given when bleeding is excluded or unlikely, has proven long-term benefit, but the effect is small (Box 2.4). Eighty patients must be treated to prevent one patient suffering death or dependency. If you don't treat the patient in front of you, he or she is unlikely to come to much harm. However, applied across the UK to, say, 60 000 suitable ischaemic stroke patients per year, 750 will be saved from death or dependency.
- Give aspirin 150–300 mg orally or rectally, thereafter 75 mg per day orally (or 300 mg rectally), except where chances of haemorrhage are clinically thought to be high (loss of consciousness, headache, vomiting).

Anticoagulation

Anticoagulation is unlikely to be beneficial in most acute strokes, including those associated with atrial fibrillation (Box 2.4). In some situations anticoagulation is sensible, including:
- An under-anticoagulated patient with a mechanical heart valve.
- Vertebral or carotid arterial dissection.
- Basilar artery thrombosis.
- Venous sinus thrombosis.

Anticoagulation with heparin (5000 IU IV, then 15–25 IU/kg per h, and check APTT after 4–6 h then daily, or 4–6 h after a dose change) is more reversible than LMWHs, so might be safer if there is bleeding. LMWHs (e.g. enoxaparin) are more convenient and less prone to under- or over-coagulation. There is no hard evidence to guide the choice.

Basilar artery thrombosis has a poor prognosis if untreated. If symptoms are progressing, and a basilar artery thrombosis has been demonstrated radiologically, consider intra-arterial thrombolysis if there is sufficient local expertise (interventional neuroradiologists). Some case series suggest that mortality is halved (to about 40%) by thrombolysis. Intervention can be up to 12 h or more from stroke onset. Otherwise anticoagulate with heparin. By the time progression has reached coma and quadriparesis, survival is unlikely.

Low-dose heparin (5000 IU bd SC), or prophylactic dose LMWH, prevents DVTs, but does not alter outcomes overall. Consider it for patients at very high risk (e.g. immobile and a history of venous thromboembolism, or severely overweight). Otherwise use compression stockings, aspirin, and early mobilization to reduce risk.

Box 2.4 International Stroke Trial (IST) and Chinese Acute Stroke Trial (CAST)

- IST: 20 000 patients with acute stroke (within 48 h) randomized patients to aspirin 300 mg/day or placebo, and heparin (25 000 IU/day or 10 000 IU/day) or placebo, in a 2 x 2 factorial design, for 14 days, or discharge if sooner.

- CAST: 21 100 patients randomized to 160 mg/day of aspirin or placebo for 4 weeks or until discharged.

- *Aspirin*: small reduction in risk of death, dependency or recurrent stroke. In IST deaths within 14 days were 9.0% vs. 9.4% (risk ratio 0.96); death or recurrent strokes were 11.3% vs. 12.4% (risk ratio 0.91); death or dependency at 6 months were 62.2% vs. 63.5% (risk ratio 0.98). No subgroup benefited significantly more or less. In CAST deaths were 3.9% vs. to 3.3% (risk ratio 0.85); death or non-fatal stroke 5.9% vs. 5.3% (risk ratio 0.89); death or dependency 31.6% vs. 30.5% (risk ratio 0.97). Pooled odds ratios for death or non-fatal stroke were 0.89 (95% CI 0.83–0.95), and for death or dependency were 0.95 (95% CI 0.91–0.99) in favour of aspirin treatment. There was a small excess of cerebral bleeds on aspirin (1.01% vs. 0.83%).

- *Heparin*: no difference in the number of deaths within 14 days—9.0% vs. 9.3% (risk ratio 0.97); and death or dependency at 6 months was 62.9% in each group. Fewer recurrent ischaemic strokes were balanced by an increase in haemorrhagic strokes. The lower dose of heparin was associated with fewer deaths and non-fatal strokes than the higher dose, but there was no advantage in the death or dependence end-point at 6 months. No subgroup, including 3000 patients with atrial fibrillation, benefited significantly more than the average.

Lancet 1997; **349**: 1569–81, 1641–9

Acute management of intracerebral haemorrhage

- Primary brain damage from the bleed will be complete and irreversible almost immediately.
- Treatment aimed at limiting neurological damage tries to prevent secondary damage, which is largely ischaemic due to local pressure reducing tissue perfusion.
- Logically evacuation of the haematoma should help, but the one large trial of this found no benefit. Conservative management is reasonable, but neurosurgeons may attempt evacuation, especially in a younger patient, with a superficial bleed and no more than moderate depression of consciousness, when an underlying aneurysm is suspected, or when an initially well patient is deteriorating.
- Cerebellar haematoma is an exception, where evacuation may be life-saving and the prospects for good functional recovery are reasonable.
- Prognosis is poor when consciousness is lost, and hopeless if there is no response to pain and absent brainstem reflexes for a few hours.
- The mainstay of treatment, as with cerebral infarcts, is to optimize brain perfusion and oxygenation by supporting cardiorespiratory function (oxygen, fluids to maintain BP), limiting other damaging physiological abnormalities (pyrexia, hyperglycaemia), and preventing or aggressively treating systemic complications.
- There is no evidence to support reducing high BP, but at very high levels (>220/110) some doctors feel modest lowering (25%, or no lower than 180/100) may help. The greater danger is from low BP compromising cerebral perfusion.

Anticoagulated patients with intracerebral haemorrhage

- The risk of bleeding to life and health outweighs the risk from clotting in the short term.
- Consult a haematologist urgently:
  - If on warfarin—reverse the anticoagulation with prothrombin complex concentrate (factors II, VII, IX, and X; 'beriplex'® 50 u/kg IV, or fresh frozen plasma 15 ml/kg IV) plus 10 mg vitamin K IV.
  - If on heparin, stop infusion. Reverse with protamine sulphate (1 mg/100U heparin received in last 3 h; initial 10 mg test dose IV over 10 min, observe for anaphylaxis; if stable give entire calculated dose slowly over 10 min; maximum dose 50 mg). A lower dose is needed as time from heparin administration increases e.g. half dose only 30 min after infusion stopped.
  - If on LMWH (e.g. enoxaparin, dalteparin), only 60% of anti-Xa activity is reversed by protamine. There is no other antidote.
  - If thrombolysed, give fibrinogen concentrate (or cryoprecipitate), and platelets (if <100 x 10^9/l). Check fibrinogen level, if <1 g/l give more. Antifibrinolytics (aprotinin or tranexamic acid) probably don't help.
  - Factor VIII if haemophiliac.
  - Platelets if thrombocytopenic (<80 x 10^9/l).
- If the patient has a mechanical heart valve, it is safe to discontinue anticoagulation for 2 weeks, both for aortic and mitral valves.

How long for?

Continue physiological normalization until the patient is stable. With minor strokes, aggressive IV therapy may not be required at all. Patients with moderate or severe strokes are unstable (i.e. liable to deteriorate) over a week or more. Judge each patient's needs day to day depending on the circumstances. Generally we suggest continuing supportive measures for 2–7 days.

Acute nursing care

Recognize two complimentary roles, one or other of which may predominate, but which often go on together:

- Supportive, active, 'doing for' care, in severe acute illness.
- Encouraging, enabling, progressive withdrawal of support to promote independence.

This section concentrates on the acute supportive role.

Maintain airway

Nurse in the coma position if unconscious. An oral airway or intubation may be necessary.

Maintain oxygenation

- The ultimate size of the infarct may depend on maintaining adequate oxygen delivery to the ischaemic brain.
- Monitor oxygen saturation by pulse oximetry. Aim to keep saturation >95%. Give 28% oxygen (2–4 l/min) by mask or nasal cannulae, if necessary, unless contraindicated.
- Stop oxygen and call for medical reassessment if respiratory rate drops below 10/min, or if desaturation (<90%) occurs on oxygen (indicating that respiratory drive may be dependent on hypoxia, sometimes seen in chronic obstructive pulmonary disease).

Avoid pressure sores

- These can arise in as little as 30 min when a severely immobile patient is placed on a sufficiently hard surface. They can develop in accident and emergency and radiology departments, as well as on wards. Vulnerable sites are the sacrum, greater trochanters, and heels. Sores are painful, debilitating, and unpleasant. A deep sore can take many months to heal, consuming expensive materials and scarce nursing time.
- Complete a pressure sore risk score immediately on admission, and certainly within 4 h (e.g. Waterlow). Most sores are avoidable with sufficient attention to pressure relief. Avoidance by turning alone is labour intensive.
- Pressure relieving mattresses (and cushions for chairs) should be immediately available 24 h/day. These cannot prevent all sores, and a turning regime is also required. Additional attention is needed to prevent heel sores.
- Reassess risk every 24 h.

Hydration and nutrition

- Swallowing is not safe initially in about half of stroke patients admitted to hospital. Nurses (and doctors) should be able to make a simple assessment of whether swallowing is safe or not. The patient must be sitting up, and conscious level sufficient to allow co-operation.
  - give a sip (5–10 ml) of water;
  - observe for failure to seal the lips;
  - look/feel for prompt laryngeal elevation indicating swallowing;
  - record if it is delayed or incomplete;

- observe for choking, coughing, or a 'wet' quality to the voice, indicating fluid around the vocal cords;
- if all appears well, repeat twice, and then try a larger volume;
- then observe while eating their first meal for coughing or choking, chewing problems, loss of food from lips, or inability to move food in the mouth (pouching);
- at the same time check for mouth dryness or other mouth care needs.
- You cannot swallow with your neck extended. Positioning is therefore very important—sitting up, or leaning slightly forward.
- If swallowing is not safe:
  - do not give anything by mouth;
  - make plans for mouth care;
  - hydrate IV, and consider nasogastric feeding;
  - repeat the swallow assessment at least daily;
  - refer to a speech and language therapist if still unsafe on days 2–3, and the patient is alert and well enough to co-operate.
- IV hydration may also be required to maintain an optimal BP (systolic pressure >140 mmHg).
- Nasogastric tubes:
  - use one if oral intake is inadequate by day 2, so long as death is not thought to be imminent, and your best information is that the patient would have wanted you to do so;
  - you may need one earlier, e.g. to administer medication;
  - many people find these uncomfortable or irritating, and they are often dislodged or pulled out;
  - they also disrupt oesophageal peristalsis and cardiac sphincter function, are associated with gastro-oesophageal reflux and increase the risk of aspiration;
  - however, they can deliver adequate nutrition in many cases.

Antivenous thrombosis prophylaxis

- If the patient is not able to walk, apply full-length compression stockings (to both legs) unless there is suspicion of arterial insufficiency.
- Check for a history of peripheral vascular disease or diabetes, and for ulcers, foot pulses, and capillary return. If in doubt, measure the ankle to brachial BP ratio (using a Doppler machine: <0.8 indicates arterial disease). Be careful if the patient has loss of sensation in the feet.
- Measure the legs for correct fit. Do not allow the stocking tops to roll and constrict the legs, as this impedes venous return.
- Check the legs and feet daily, and change stockings every 3 days.
- Continue until the patient is mobile.
- Aspirin, good hydration, and early mobilization all help prevent DVTs in addition.
- Low-dose heparin (5000 IU bd SC), or prophylactic dose LMWH, prevents DVTs, but does not alter outcomes overall. Consider it if patient is at very high risk (e.g. immobile and a history of venous thromboembolism, or severe overweight), or if compression stocking are contraindicated.

Positioning and support

A positioning and handling plan is required as part of the initial nursing and physiotherapy assessments.

- The aim of early intervention is:
  - to prevent abnormal tone, contractures and pressure sores;
  - to maintain correct alignment of body parts to make normal movement patterns possible or easier;
  - to avoid the establishment of abnormal patterns.
- Distinguish between:
  - comfort positioning (for agitated or dying patients);
  - therapeutic positioning (which maximizes the chances of future recovery and function).
- Prolonged supine lying increases extensor spasticity and should be avoided unless comfort is the priority:
  - place a pillow under the head and affected shoulder.
  - legs should lie symmetrically.
- Side lying is preferred (Figures 2.1 and 2.2):
  - support the head on one pillow;
  - the trunk should be straight;
  - bring the hemiplegic arm out in front of the patient, extended if underneath, slightly flexed if on top;
  - make sure the shoulder is forward so that the weight is slightly behind the shoulder tip;
  - extend the hemiplegic leg, and flex the unaffected leg to give support—*don't* support under the foot (to dorsiflex it), as this can stimulate extensor activity;
  - support the upper arm, leg, and back with pillows.

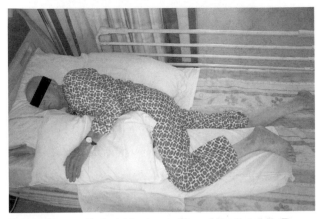

Fig. 2.1 Correct positioning, left hemiparesis, lying on the unaffected side. The trunk is straight. The shoulder is forward and the hemiplegic arm in front of the patient. The hemiplegic leg is extended. The head, trunk and upper arm are supported by pillows.

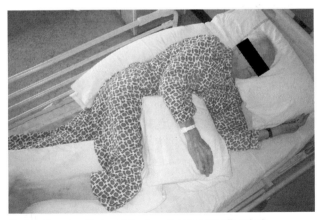

Fig. 2.2 Correct positioning, left hemiparesis, lying on the affected side.

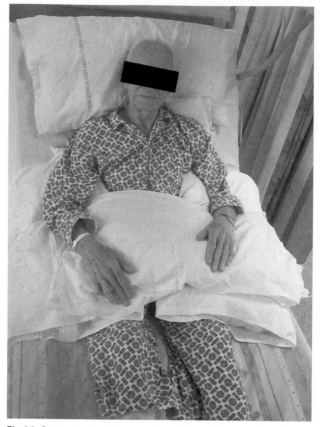

Fig. 2.3 Correct positioning, sitting in bed (e.g. for feeding). The trunk is upright and symmetrical, supported on both sides, a pillow under the affected arm. There is additional support behind the affected shoulder.

- If sitting in bed (Figure 2.3):
  - keep upright and symmetrical;
  - supported on both sides;
  - a pillow under the hemiplegic forearm.

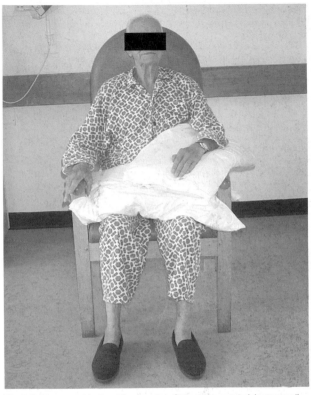

Fig. 2.4 Correct positioning, sitting in a chair. Sitting is symmetrical, bottom well back in the chair. Feet are flat on the floor. The hip, knees and ankle are at right angles, and well aligned. Affected arm is supported on a pillow.

- When sitting in a chair (Figure 2.4):
  - the hip, knees, and ankle should be at right angles;
  - feet flat on the floor;
  - keep the hip well-aligned, as it will tend to fall into external rotation;
  - sitting should be symmetrical (equal weight on each buttock);
  - support the trunk on both sides with pillows or rolled towels, or use specialist trunk supports or chairs (e.g. Wolfston, Hydrotilt) to keep the patient relaxed;
  - the paralysed arm should be supported on a pillow, placed forward (shoulder slightly flexed), close to the trunk, and in neutral rotation or slightly externally rotated, with the elbow in neutral flexion/extension.

The affected shoulder

Take care with it. Damage may be done very early on. Shoulder pain can be very persistent.

- There is often insufficient muscle activity to support the joint in its correct position. Incorrect handling can sublux the joint and damage the joint capsule.
- When the patient is sitting:
  - support the arm with a pillow to keep the humerus in a neutral position and close to the body;
  - keep the wrist and fingers straight;
  - don't ignore an arm hanging over the side of the bed or chair.
- Support the arm under the shoulder when moving it away from the body, and limit movement away from the body to 30° at most.
- Encourage the patient to hold or support his or her own arm at the wrist when transferring or standing.
- When lying on the affected side, ease the shoulder forward so the patient's weight is slightly behind the shoulder tip.
- Never pull on the affected arm.
- Encourage active movement.
- Discourage gripping activities (they promote abnormal tone).

Transferring

The primary aim is to avoid injuries to the patient (shoulder, falls) and staff (back and neck), which have been unfortunately common in the past. Transferring is also a therapeutic opportunity.

- Like all practical physical skills, you cannot learn this from a book. You need proper training and supervised practice.
- A manual handling assessment should be made as soon as possible after admission, and certainly within 12 h.
  - take account of alertness, communication, cognition, vision, and previous ability;
  - you must have access to appropriate transferring aids;
  - if there is doubt about safety, a physiotherapist should assess and advise.
- The transfer will not work unless the patient can stand safely, and can engage in active co-operation.
- Use an aid if the transfer is difficult. If in doubt, always choose the safer option.
- Beware a patient who tries to grab you as he or she stands.
- A patient who pushes to one side during a transfer is likely to slip or overbalance.
- If necessary, use a hoist. It will do the job, but is slow and non-therapeutic.
- A standing hoist encourages some standing.
- A rotunda involves standing, but encourages overuse of the unaffected side, and poor-quality standing alignment.
- 'Banana' (sliding) boards can be used for (sitting) bed–chair transfers, and encourage participation.
- Transfer with a Zimmer or rollator frame only after a physiotherapy assessment.

Bladder and bowel management

- 60% of patients admitted with stroke will be initially incontinent of urine.
- An early assessment of the likely cause of incontinence should always be made including:
  - dipstick urinalysis;
  - postvoid residual volume (by ultrasound or catheterization);
  - ascertaining previous bladder and bowel problems.
- Indwelling urethral catheters always cause problems, including infection, blockage, bladder spasm, and urethral trauma. They are best avoided:
  - if there is retention, intermittent catheterization is preferable;
  - a sheath catheter or incontinence pads should be able to keep the skin dry, and contain wetness adequately;
  - however, for patients with drowsiness, severe immobility, absent sitting balance, or developing skin problems, it is hard to argue that a catheter is never an acceptable means of containment in the short term, so long as the decision is constantly reviewed.

Explanation and reassurance

The patient is likely to be frightened and bewildered, especially if dysphasic. Relatives may be as well.

Monitoring

Monitoring should be:
- Tailored to meet the circumstances of the individual patient.
- Reviewed regularly, so scarce nursing and medical time is not wasted with unnecessary observations.
- Prioritized—it may be necessary to compromise on the ideal, if other important tasks (rehabilitation nursing, counselling) are neglected because of time spent on 'monitoring'.

A thrombolysed patient requires high-dependency monitoring (Appendix 7). Otherwise, the following parameters should be considered acutely:
- Neurological status:
  - level of consciousness—the Glasgow Coma Scale (Appendix 3) is well-established and familiar, and changes of more than three points, or a gradually declining score require explanation and/or action;
  - progression of neurological impairments—this can be by serial traditional neurological examination, or using a stroke severity scale, such as the Scandinavian or National Institutes of Health (NIH) stroke scales (Appendices 8 and 9).
- Cardiovascular status: pulse and BP, 4 hourly initially. May be required more often if unstable.
- Respiratory: respiratory rate and pulse oximetry.
- Temperature.
- Blood glucose (by glucometer), if diabetic or initially raised and/or on hypoglycaemic drugs.
- Food and fluid intake.

Appendix 4 is a care pathway directing early monitoring.

Involving therapists

- In a well-organized acute stroke ward, there should be no need for specific referral of patients to therapists by doctors.
- Rehabilitation should start as soon as the patient is able, and this is best assessed daily between therapists and nurses. This may be on day 1.
- Early mobilization is a key feature of specialized stroke unit care.
- Highly successful Scandinavian stroke services describe very aggressive early mobilization even for very severely affected patients (physiotherapist assessment within 6 h, out of bed within 24 h).
- For less severely affected patients this will allow early functional mobility or discharge.
- For others, it reduces the chances of venous thrombosis and other complications of immobility. However, it must be safe (avoiding falls, shoulder problems and injuries to staff), and should not promote abnormal tone, or adversely affect potential for recovery of normal movement patterns.
- Early mobilization is labour intensive. Transferring and standing a hemiplegic patient can take two or more therapists. Mechanical aids (hoists, standing hoists) must be available.
- Physiotherapists will sometimes see unconscious or very ill patients, predominantly to advise on positioning (mainly to improve lung ventilation).
- OTs' rapid assessment of minimally disabled patients may help early discharge. Otherwise basic assessment can be undertaken if the patient is sufficiently alert, including perceptual and cognitive screening, and ascertaining previous functional and social information.
- Patients with impaired swallowing on initial screening, or communication problems, should be referred to a speech and language therapist, but this can wait a day or two.

Communication

- Good communication is primarily a matter of common courtesy. But adequate explanation may also help reduce anxiety and psychological distress, in both patients and family members. A policy of proactive information giving may reduce complaints.
- Communication may be difficult, because of drowsiness, dysphasia, or confusion. Patients often forget what they are told, especially if anxious in the presence of doctors. Explanations may have to be repeated several times.
- Don't assume that all family members get on or share information, although it can be pointed out to them that it helps hard-pressed medical and nursing staff if they can be seen together, or a key-contact person is appointed who will pass on what they are told.
- Patients and their families will need an explanation of:
  - what a stroke is;
  - what the process of care in hospital will be (whether admission is necessary, what follow-up arrangements are if not, where they will be admitted to, what tests or treatment is likely);
  - what the immediate prognosis is (stroke may be life threatening, what good or bad signs there are);
  - when more information will be available.
- Some immediate decision making may be required, that should ideally involve information from, or to, families (e.g. resuscitation).
- Let nursing and medical colleagues know what the diagnosis is, and what your plans are (especially if you are not going to have ongoing responsibility). Best done by writing it clearly in the case notes.

Summary

1. Most patients should be admitted to hospital, unless they are minimally disabled and can be assessed and investigated as an out-patient within a week.
2. In hospital, on day 1 you need to make or confirm the diagnosis of stroke, order initial investigations, and instigate plans for relief of pressure areas, feeding and hydration, maintaining oxygenation, and bladder and bowel management.
3. Some stroke patients are very ill, and require careful nursing, with particular regard to swallowing, pressure areas, positioning, continence, and care of the unconscious patient.
4. Initial medical management of cerebral infarcts involves hydration and aspirin. There are likely benefits from a more intensive regimen of physiological monitoring, manipulation of BP to achieve moderate hypertension, and correction in abnormalities in oxygenation, hyperglycaemia, and pyrexia.
5. Suitably equipped and trained units may consider thrombolysis for carefully selected patients with ischaemic strokes who arrive at hospital within 2 h and who can be assessed and treated within an hour.
6. Supportive management of intracerebral haemorrhage is similar, but antithrombotics must be avoided, anticoagulation or other bleeding disorders reversed, and consideration given to referral to a neurosurgeon for evacuation.
7. Neurological, respiratory, and cardiovascular function, glycaemia and temperature should be monitored closely over the first 48 h at least.
8. Let patients, relatives, and staff colleagues know what has happened and what is planned.

Chapter 3

The first two weeks

Trajectories of recovery

We can define four patterns of stroke care (excluding SAH for now):
- TIAs and minor, non-disabling stroke.
- Mildly disabling stroke, which recovers to independence within a week or two.
- Moderate or severe stroke requiring many weeks of rehabilitation to reach maximum abilities.
- Fatal stroke, requiring terminal care.

The objectives are different for each, with some overlap (Table 3.1).
- The first group will often not be admitted to hospital, or should be discharged quickly if they are. Investigation and further management should take place as an out-patient.
- The other three groups should be admitted to a specialist ward.
- We will consider terminal care separately (Chapter 7).

Table 3.1 Trajectories of stroke care

Trajectory	Objective	Action
Non-disabling	Information	Explanation and reassurance
	Aetiology	Investigation
	Secondary prevention	Carotid duplex, cardiac rhythm and function, antithrombotics, BP and cholesterol reduction, smoking cessation
	Out-patient management	Refer to specialist clinic
Minor disabling	Information	Explanation and reassurance
	Aetiology	Investigation
	Secondary prevention	As for non-disabling stroke
	Functional assessment/ rehabilitation	Nursing, SLT, OT, and physiotherapy
	Rapid discharge	Accessing community rehabilitation and follow-up services
Moderate–severe disabling	Diagnosis	Review by expert clinician
	Survival	Physiological support, nursing care
	Avoidance of complications	Expert nursing and medical care
	Securing hydration and nutrition	Monitor swallowing, IV, nasogastrically, or gastrostomy
	Rehabilitation	Nursing, SLT, OT, and physiotherapy on a dedicated ward
Fatal	Diagnosis	Review by expert clinician
	Freedom from distress	Necessary palliative treatment
	Dignity	Avoidance of unnecessary intervention

SLT, speech and language therapy.

Feeding and hydration

About half of patients admitted to hospital following a stroke cannot swallow safely. Mortality in this group is high, but the majority of survivors regain their swallowing eventually. Of those with problems initially:
• Half die within 6 weeks.
• 30% can feed orally within 2 weeks.
• Most of the rest recover safe swallowing over the next month.
• Long-term survival without safe swallowing is quite rare.

Hydration is important:
• Thirst is unpleasant, initially at least, in conscious patients before renal failure and drowsiness take over.
• Dehydration and pre-renal renal failure can develop.
• Venous thrombosis and pressure sores are more likely in dehydrated patients.
• Inadequate cardiac filling pressure may result in decreased BP, which may be harmful to the perfusion of the stroke 'penumbra'.
• Death results after 1–2 weeks with no fluid intake.

Nutrition is important:
• Hunger is unpleasant.
• Malnutrition is associated with worse outcomes and a slower rate of recovery.
• Under conditions of subnutrition, muscle is catabolized to meet metabolic needs. Resulting muscular weakness increases disability, which must be reversed during rehabilitation.
• Vitamin deficiencies or insufficiencies can occur (e.g. vitamin K increasing prothrombin time/INR, vitamin D causing myopathy and bone demineralization, especially in the face of immobility).
• Prolonged undernutrition suppresses immune function.
• Loss of 20–30% body weight results in depressed mood, which is difficult to reverse until body weight is restored.
• Wound healing (e.g. pressure sores or leg ulcers) is inhibited by poor nutrition.
• Many drugs are best given orally—there may be problems if some are omitted (e.g. for Parkinson's disease or heart failure, or those dependent on benzodiazepines).

A simple premise in clinical nutrition is that 'if there is a functioning gut, use it'. The problem in stroke care is accessing it.
Some guidelines assist safe oral feeding:
• Thickened liquids and cold, soft, single consistency foods are easier to swallow.
• You cannot swallow with your neck extended. Sit the patient up. Achieving this for someone with very poor trunk control is not easy, and can be labour intensive.
• Risk of aspiration can be reduced by flexing the neck ('a chin tuck') before swallowing (this closes the airway and opens the gullet).
• Pacing—take it slowly, allow time for each mouthful to be cleared before giving another. Some patients 'pouch' food in their cheeks if they cannot swallow it. This needs removing (with a drink or a finger) at the end of the meal.

If, despite these measures, swallowing is unsafe by day 2, consider nasogastric feeding. Mouth care and monitoring for recovery of swallowing should continue.

If oral intake is inadequate after about 2–3 weeks consider gastrostomy feeding:

- The practicalities of PEG insertion are listed in Table 3.2. It takes a few days to think about and organize.
- They do not cause discomfort (after the first couple of days), are difficult to dislodge, and can be managed in rehabilitation hospitals or at home.
- They do not suffer the same problems with reflux seen with nasogastric tubes.
- The procedure is under local anaesthetic with midazolam sedation. Removal may require a further endoscopy.
- If the patient is not fit for endoscopy, or there are other reasons why this is technically difficult, radiological insertion ('RIG', with ultrasound or fluoroscopy guidance) is possible.

If swallowing ability is recovering, but not yet safe or adequate for nutrition by 2 weeks it can be difficult to judge whether to proceed to gastrostomy or not. Waiting another week or so is reasonable.

A standardized tube-feeding regimen can be used initially. Refer to a dietician for assessment of individualized nutrition requirements and an appropriate feed prescription.

Videofluoroscopy may be required where 'silent aspiration' is suspected.

Table 3.2 Practical issues surrounding gastrostomy tube insertion

Issue	Action
Peri-procedure mortality is about 1%	Inform patient and/or family
Desirability	Full information and counselling required
Consent	Formal consent necessary, best interest declaration if lacking capacity
Clotting (may be deranged after starvation)	Check FBC, INR, and APTT. Give vitamin K if necessary
Dehydration	Check electrolytes and renal function, correct IV if necessary
Respiratory function—dangerous desaturation can occur during endoscopy	Optimize. Postpone if active chest infection. Consider radiological placement.
Previous gastric surgery, severe obesity	Consult endoscopist. Consider radiological placement
If prolonged starvation or severe malnutrition, possible re-feeding syndrome (rhabdomyolysis, heart and respiratory failure, arrhythmias, seizures)	Give thiamine, start feed slowly, monitor serum phosphate, potassium, magnesium, and calcium for first 4 days. If phosphate less than 0.5 mmol/l, give IV phosphate 50 mmol over 24 h

Neurological problems

Hemiparesis

- Weakness may affect the face, arm, or leg, or a more limited part such as the hand.
- The extent of paralysis may deteriorate in the first week, probably as the ischaemic penumbra infarcts. No proven intervention can avert this (apart from early aspirin, to a small extent). Measures to optimize physiology (BP, oxygenation, blood glucose, temperature) probably help. Anticoagulation doesn't improve outcome overall.
- Resistance to passive movement (tone), reflecting resting muscle activity, is often low initially, but may be normal, and it can increase over subsequent days or weeks (spasticity may develop).
- Cortical infarcts (TACI and PACI) typically affect the arm more than the leg. This is because the motor cortex supplying the leg derives its blood supply partly from the anterior cerebral artery (rather than the middle cerebral artery).
- Isolated anterior cerebral artery infarcts (the leg is affected and the arm spared) are uncommon—review the diagnosis.
- Subcortical infarcts (lacunar strokes, affecting the internal capsule or brainstem tracts) can result in a dense, flaccid, paralysis of both arm and leg equally.

Recovery of hemiparesis is a combination of three things:

- Spontaneous recovery.
- Active therapy.
- Avoidance of complications.

Spontaneous recovery accounts for the greater part. Increasing evidence suggests that active therapy is important to maximize and make use of the recovery, without developing or reinforcing dysfunctional, abnormal movements.

- If paralysis is severe, initial management tries to re-establish head and trunk stability using therapeutic positioning and limb support, to achieve sitting, independence in eating, and upper body self-care.
- Early muscle use stimulates neuroplasticity and normal muscular activation, e.g. sitting and standing help develop trunk control.
- Early standing promotes muscle activation through weight bearing, provides sensory feedback, and improves alertness, pressure area care, bowel function, and morale.
- Early training in functional tasks (e.g. transfers) makes handling easier, and reduces the chances of complications.
- The patient is taught to minimize compensatory tactics and overuse of the unaffected side. This encourages activity on the affected side, and avoids reinforcement of abnormal movement patterns.
- Encourage active use of a weak but functional arm to maintain sensory and proprioceptive input, and minimize muscle atrophy.
- Therapists gradually 'progress' activity, and use a teaching approach to promote 'carry over' between sessions. The emphasis is on relearning normal movement patterns that can be built upon.
- These principles must be continued throughout the 24-h period to maximize effect, so nurses must be familiar with the moving and handling plan, in consultation with physiotherapists.

Dysphasia (or aphasia)

The experience of dysphasia has been compared with (a non-Russian speaker) travelling on the Moscow Metro. You know where you want to go, and may want to ask a fellow traveller where to get off, but you can't make yourself understood. You can see the signs at the stations but cannot understand what they mean.

There are a dozen or more subtypes of dysphasia. They boil down to:
- Problems with expression.
- Problems with understanding.
- Both together (mixed).

Relatives (and some non-specialist staff) may think the patient has become confused. They may respond by treating him or her as if they had.
- Doctors, nurses, and therapists should discuss functional communication (expression and understanding).
- Explain repeatedly to the patient, and relatives, the nature of the problem.
- Empathize—imagine what it would be like if it happened to you (one day in several decades time it may). You would find life frustrating, possibly unbearably so. You probably wouldn't understand what was going on. You would wonder if you were going to recover, but might fear that you would not. Lack of communication ability may lead you to be incontinent, thirsty, or in pain. Co-operation with therapy may be hard, and you might be thought to be difficult or unmotivated.
- Assume that understanding is retained, even when expression is severely affected. Explain that the stroke disconnected the thinking bit of the brain from the speaking bit (or disconnected the hearing bit from the understanding bit). Explain the same to family members.
- Encourage visitors not to give up, give the patient time to get things out, and use language as much as possible with the patient.

What to do:
- Get an early speech and language therapy assessment and advice on non-verbal communication, for both staff and relatives.
- Keep language simple. No long or obscure words. Short sentences. One idea at a time. No double negatives. Avoid medical jargon.
- Give plenty of time.
- Use gesture, and symbols or pictures.
- The disorder is of language rather than speaking, so written communication will usually be affected also. In any case, usually the patient's writing hand will be affected. But it is worth writing things down to see if it helps.

Speech and language therapists are experts in communication, and strategies to get round problems. High-intensity therapy targeted at specific aspects of language function improves communication. In addition, therapists have a wider role in advising, counselling, and supporting the relatives of people with dysphasia.

OTs use an alternative approach. Practising familiar functional tasks (e.g. washing and dressing) allows engagement and rehabilitation of trunk and upper limbs without the patient being necessarily able to follow instructions.

Emotional lability or emotionalism

- This is emotional expression (usually crying, rarely laughing) that is inappropriate to (or extreme for) the emotional context.
- It is not the same as depression, but is disabling and distressing to the patient (and those around them).
- Develops (in 15%) over the first week or two.
- Degrees of severity can be defined by the emotional content of triggers (usually spoken statements) that bring on the crying.
- Examine the mental state further, as depression (major affective disorder) is also a cause of crying.
- Explain the problem to patient and relatives.
- Usually responds within a few days to SSRIs (fluoxetine 20 mg od) or tricyclic antidepressants (lofepramine 70 mg at night or bd, dothiepin starting at 50–75 mg at night)—much quicker than you would expect for depression.
- Tends to resolve or improve over time.

Neglect (Table 3.3)

Unawareness or relative disregard of one side of the world is a feature of parietal lobe damage, typically, but not exclusively, when the non-dominant side is affected. If it occurs with dominant parietal lobe lesions, assessment is often complicated by communication problems. It may be transient or persisting, and lesser degrees are often missed.

- Do not confuse with hemianopia (which may also cause problems with perception on one side, but which is more easily compensated by moving the point of visual fixation).
- Can be a major barrier to rehabilitation and recovery.
- Needs looking for explicitly. Doctors, nurses, and therapists may all help in recognizing it.
- Pencil and paper tests, more formal 'parietal lobe batteries', or neuropsychological assessment can be used. Tests include Albert's test (line cancellation), clock face drawing, or drawing double-headed flowers.
- Spontaneous recovery is more important than specific therapy.
- Reduce isolation by positioning (with respect to walls etc.) so that the non-neglected side is facing the world. An older fashion for 'forcing' use of the neglectful side by doing the converse was not helpful.
- Explain it to relatives—as with all bizarre and unusual phenomena.

Other features of parietal lobe dysfunction

- Astereognosis—inability to recognize objects placed in the affected hand.
- Agraphaesthesia—inability to recognize a number drawn (with the examiner's finger) on the palm of the patient's hand.
- Geographical disorientation—inability to navigate, or gets lost in, familiar surroundings, despite the ability to see.
- Dressing apraxia—inability to dress (or perform other purposeful constructional tasks) in the absence of weakness, sensory or visual loss, or neglect that would explain it. May occur in a pure form.

Table 3.3 Aspects of neglect

Feature	Description
Visual extinction	Failure to register a stimulus such as finger movement in the periphery of a visual field, when a similar, simultaneous, stimulus is applied to the opposite side
Sensory extinction	Failure to register a tactile stimulus such as hand touching, when a similar, simultaneous, stimulus is applied to the opposite side
Topographical neglect	Neglect during drawing, copying, constructional tasks, line cancellation or bisection
Hemi-inattention	Behaviour during clinical examination or therapy suggesting inability to respond to environmental stimuli on one side (noises, people approaching)
Anosognosia	Denial of the presence of neurological deficit such as weakness. Can result in falls and fractures if the patient confidently tries to walk on a paralysed leg.
Denial of body parts	Denial of ownership, lack of awareness of a limb
Anosodiasphoria	Lack of concern for the neurological deficit

Persisting drowsiness

Most patients who are initially drowsy either die or recover in the first week or two. A few patients who remain drowsy are especially problematic. They are not fit enough to engage in therapy, and appear to be in 'limbo'.
- Exclude metabolic, infective and drug causes.
- Consider hydrocephalus and recurrent stroke—repeat the CT scan.
- The patient may be terminally ill, and a decision to withdraw active or supportive treatments may need to be taken.
- Some patients have prolonged periods of drowsiness or sleeping, and be fairly well during the few hours they are awake. Dexamphetamine (5 mg od, increasing every few days up to 60 mg/day) or modafinil (100 mg od increasing up to bd, morning and noon, or 200 mg bd) is worth trying. Watch for hypertension and fits. L-dopa is also sometimes tried.

Neurological deterioration

A common reason for requesting a medical review is because of neurological deterioration (Table 3.4). It may occur at any time. This may be:
- Decreased level of consciousness.
- Fitting.
- Worsening focal neurological signs.

Trans-tentorial herniation is the commonest cause of death in the first week. It generally:
- Occurs within 24 h of bleeds.
- Peaks at days 4–5 after infarction (due to oedema formation).

Haemorrhagic transformation occurs in 75% of cardioembolic strokes, and 30% of all infarcts, within 4 days. Neurological deterioration occurs in 20% of these.

Table 3.4 Neurological deterioration after stroke

Cause	Action
'Evolving' stroke—worsening symptoms over 24 h or so.	Review diagnosis, early CT scan. Anticoagulation is not indicated.
Raised intracranial pressure/herniation (oedema), hydrocephalus	Repeat CT scan. In the UK, mostly just observation. Consider mannitol or neurosurgical opinion.
Recurrent stroke	Seek 'active' embolic source (e.g. cardiac, including endocarditis), alternative diagnosis, e.g. vasculitis or fits. Otherwise manage as first stroke.
Haemorrhagic transformation of infarct	Stop aspirin or anticoagulants.
Intercurrent infection	Check white cell count and inflammatory markers, review especially chest and urine.
Drug adverse effect	Review
Metabolic disturbance	Check glucose, electrolytes (SIADH in 10% of strokes).
Fitting (about 5% in acute phase)	Clinical diagnosis, need eye witness account. Likely to recur if after the first 24 h. Oral sodium valproate is antiepileptic drug of choice, or IV phenytoin if no oral access.

Medical problems

Hypertension

- BP goes up after a stroke, and comes down again over the next week.
- Initial BP is related to outcome (fatality is least in those with initial systolic pressures between 140 and 180 mmHg), but it is unclear if any manipulations, up or down, improve outcomes.
- Unless there is evidence of immediate end-organ damage (encephalopathy, heart or renal failure) or other hypertensive emergency, do not give antihypertensive drugs for at least a week.
- As far as we know at present, BP reduction is primarily a longer-term (months to years) secondary preventative intervention, so there is no hurry.
- However, it is logistically convenient to start establishing a secondary prevention regimen while the patient is in hospital.
- After the first week, the ward BP record makes a good assessment of 'usual' BP.
- Start with bendrofluazide/bendroflumethazide 2.5 mg od, and add an ACE inhibitor (any will probably do, e.g. perindopril 2–4 mg od, or enalapril 5–20 mg od), unless there are strong contraindications, or indications for using something else. See Chapter 10.

Hyperglycaemia

- If glucose is raised initially, it will often also come down of its own accord (a 'stress' response).
- There is moderate evidence (observational level, cohort studies) that initially raised glucose is associated with poorer outcomes. There is a plausible biological mechanism to explain this (glucose metabolism in ischaemic brain may be cytotoxic).
- Therefore, raised glucose should be reduced (insulin sliding scale) to keep the blood sugar under 10 mmol/l. These are labour intensive, and need a lot of finger-prick monitoring, so can be converted rapidly to a twice-daily insulin regimen (isophane or isophane/soluble mix) very quickly.
- If requirements are low, and oral feeding has been re-established, try withdrawing therapy, or converting to oral hypoglycaemics after a week.
- Remember the longer-term objectives of diabetes management:
  • avoidance of symptoms (thirst, polyuria, pruritis);
  • avoidance of diabetic crises (hypoglycaemia, ketoacidosis, and non-ketotic hyperosmolar coma);
  • avoidance of (micro)vascular complications in the longer term.
- The newly diagnosed diabetic will need a strategic plan. The symptoms most likely to cause problems are polyuria and nocturia—especially if the stroke has left the bladder unstable and mobility uncertain. In the diagnosed diabetic, especially if elderly and frail, hypoglycaemia is more likely to be a problem than hyperglycaemic states. Moderately tight control should be the goal—pre-meal blood glucose measurements between 5 and 12 mmol/l.

- Maintaining euglycaemia is a relatively ineffective way of avoiding (macro)vascular complications. The vast majority of this group will be at high vascular risk and should be offered the full range of vascular preventative measures.
- Diabetic complications may complicate rehabilitation, including retinopathy and cataract, peripheral vascular disease, peripheral neuropathy (compromises balance), and neuropathic and ischaemic foot ulcers.
- An admission for stroke is an opportunity to ensure that comprehensive screening for diabetic complications is performed (dilated fundoscopy, renal function and proteinuria, test sensation, foot care).

Medical complications

A 'complication' is a secondary disease or condition aggravating a previous one. Stroke care is medically active—50% or more of patients develop medical complications.

It is useful to distinguish between:

- Neurological features of the initial stroke, such as spasticity, dysphagia, neglect, or fitting.
- Effects of recurrent stroke, or other coincidental vascular events (e.g. heart attack).
- Effects of pre-existing, comorbid, conditions (e.g. arthritis, or dementia).
- 'True' complications—new conditions arising because of the stroke.
- Associated medical conditions—such as high BP, hyperglycaemia.

All of these increase the complexity of managing stroke. Each problem needs to be managed carefully and optimally, to ensure the best chance of a good outcome.

'True complications' are dominated by the effects of immobility, and psychological responses (Table 3.5).

Chest infections result from aspiration, drowsiness, and immobility. Urinary infections are usually catheter associated, but are common in elderly women in any case.

DVTs:

- Develop in 50% of patients with a hemiplegia, but are usually subclinical.
- Clinically apparent DVT occurs in about 5%.
- Clinically important pulmonary emboli occur in 1–2%, but are common at post mortem in patients who die after 2–4 weeks.
- Early LMWH or anticoagulation prevents DVT, but appears to have little impact on overall outcome.
- Aspirin is also an effective venous antithrombotic.
- Full-length compression stockings are widely used, and are sensible, if unproven.

Table 3.5 True complications of stroke

Problem	Action
Infections	Care over feeding. Avoid urinary catheters if possible. Monitor carefully to diagnose early.
Venous thromboembolism	Hydration, early mobilization, aspirin, antiembolism stockings. Prophylactic LMWH if very high risk. Anticoagulant dose LMWH and warfarin for proven thromboses (or a caval filter if an intracerebral bleed).
Pressure sores	Early assessment, pressure relieving mattress and turning regime. Early mobilization.
Joint contractures	Positioning, early physiotherapy, thermoplastic splinting.
Osteoporosis	Vitamin D supplementation may help prevent. Bisphosphonate if history of low trauma fracture (see Chapter 8, section on Falls and fractures, p. 182).
Depression and anxiety	Positive therapeutic environment. Problem solving. Communication, sympathetic staff. May require antidepressant drugs, but do not rush in.
Falls and fractures	Moving and handling assessment by nurses, physiotherapists and OTs. Suitable walking aids, adequate supervision. Appropriate footwear. Minimize sedative medication. Test for postural hypotension. Bedrails (cotsides) may help or may hinder. Consider hip protectors.
Paresis or dependent oedema	Elevation (lying down, rather than footstool). Compression stockings or pneumatic boots (flowtron). Diuretics in severe cases (frusemide 20–40 mg od).
Shoulder pain or subluxation	Do not pull shoulder, or lift under arm. Careful positioning in bed and when sitting in chair. Adequate support. Physiotherapy advice. OTs assess for specialist mechanical supports. Simple analgesics, consider steroid injections.

Bladder and bowel management

Incontinence of one or both of urine and faeces is unpleasant and distressing.

- Urinary incontinence:
  - is predominantly detrusor instability (confusingly referred to as 'hyper-reflexia' when there is a neurological cause)—this recovers at the same rate as other neurological functions;
  - a proportion have incomplete bladder emptying, either caused by the stroke, or a comorbidity (most often prostatic enlargement, anticholinergic drugs, faecal impaction, or idiopathic);
  - a further proportion (perhaps a quarter) have normal bladders, but cannot communicate or move well enough to get to a toilet or urinal in time.
- Before acting, have some idea of what the diagnosis is:
  - exclude infection (dipstick, specimen for culture, if possible);
  - exclude retention (portable bladder ultrasound scanner, or residual catheter);
  - record a 48-h urine output (frequency-volume) chart.
- If the patient is dysphasic, has other communication problems or is demented, offer the toilet at least every 2 h (they may have bladder instability as well).
- Anticholinergic medication is relatively ineffective, and prone to side-effects, so should be reserved until the acute phase is over, and co-operation with a prompted voiding regime or bladder retraining is possible.
- Sometimes a catheter will be requested. If a patient can possibly be managed using incontinence pads or a sheath catheter, these should be tried. Catheters always have problems (bladder spasm with bypassing, infection, blockage, urethral trauma, stones). In one stroke unit trial, the patients on the unit had half the number of urinary infections as those on general medical wards—neatly matched by the prevalence of catheter usage.
- Use an indwelling catheter only if there is a good reason, e.g. a patient who is developing sore skin, or with incomplete bladder emptying who is difficult to catheterize or who finds intermittent catheterization distressing. Reassess the need for it regularly. Anticholinergic drugs (e.g. oxybutinin or tolterodine) can be used for catheter-induced bladder spasm.
- A care pathway is given in Appendix 10.

Managing faecal incontinence in acute stroke is difficult. Make sure the following are not responsible:

- laxatives or other drugs;
- acute diarrhoeal diseases (infections, inflammatory bowel disease);
- tube feeds;
- communication problems;
- access to toilets, commode, or bedpan;
- constipation.

Do a rectal examination to exclude impaction. An abdominal X-ray can help, if feasible. An immobile, dehydrated or undernourished person is at high risk of constipation. Primarily a stimulant laxative is required (i.e. senna—use an adequate dose, up to 30 mg or 4 tablets, or 20 ml syrup per day). If tube fed, fibre-added feeds can help. Sodium docusate (200 mg bd) is a 'wetting agent', and acts as both a softener and stimulant, and is a useful adjunct to senna. Osmotic laxatives are sometimes, but rarely, required in addition.

Other mechanisms for faecal incontinence include:
• lack of awareness
• colorectal disinhibition.

In these cases, formal bowel regimens may be useful in the longer term, but have no place in the acute phase. Containment in pads, which are changed rapidly if soiled, is probably the best option. Faecal containment bags, sometimes used on intensive care units, are a little-used alternative.

Continue to assess over time, and review for opportunities to intervene.

Starting rehabilitation

There is no clear cut-point between acute and rehabilitation phases.
- If the patient is well enough, therapy should start immediately.
- Therapy should be as intensive as possible—the maximum tolerated daily, although this is often constrained by staff availability.

Physiotherapy

- Physiotherapists should be involved early, and should make their own assessment of how much they can work with a patient.
- Early mobilization is associated with better outcomes—even after taking account of the potential confounding influence of disease severity (the least affected can mobilize sooner, and do better quite apart from their early mobility).
- If rehabilitation is to take place on a different ward from acute care, the care received should be made as seamless as possible. Type and intensity of therapy should be determined by the patient's needs not location.

Mobility related work in less severely affected patients will be undertaken by nurses and OTs as well as physiotherapists:
- They should make their own judgements about what is safe and desirable to do, but must have ready access to a physiotherapist in contentious or difficult cases.
- Delaying mobilization pending a physiotherapist's assessment indicates a poorly staffed or poorly organized system.

Occupational therapy

Early OT intervention is beneficial. Initial tasks involve:
- Assessment and information gathering, including for neglect, apraxias, and cognitive problems, which can be difficult to detect, and may have a bearing on subsequent functional tasks.
- Work on practically focused tasks such as dressing, are important morale boosters, as well as being important for discharge planning.
- Work on upper body personal care contributes to improved trunk control in patients with a severe hemiparesis.

Many day-to-day functional activities will be managed by nurses, so there must be good communication between them and other therapists. This involves:
- Understanding by nurses of what is possible and desirable in the view of therapists.
- Trust in nurses' judgement, and avoidance of overprotectiveness.
- It is possible that rehabilitation nursing, rather than any other type of therapy, makes the major difference between specialized stroke units and management on general wards.

Speech and language therapy

- Speech and language therapists spend much of their time with stroke patients dealing with swallowing problems.
- A careful interface with nursing judgement is required. Starving a patient while awaiting a speech therapy assessment may not be

necessary if *suitably trained* nurses can use their judgement in trying thickened fluids and soft foods.
• Communication assessment should not be neglected. The sudden onset of dysphasia is a distressing and bewildering experience for both patients and carers.

Documenting changes and progress

Communication is always important when a diverse group of professionals are working with a given patient.

If staff responsible for a patient change frequently, they are unlikely to get to grips with problems, cannot establish a rapport with patients or families, and may miss things. Good case notes are necessary to communicating progress, problems, and plans.

Information is required on:
- Progress of neurological impairments.
- Progress in aetiological investigation.
- Medical complications (and the evidence for them) and comorbidities.
- Discussions with the patient and family.
- Documentation of decisions made.
- Functional ability.
- Home circumstances, family or other support, prospects and progress towards discharge.

Multidisciplinary notes are sometimes used. A weekly team meeting should be convened and thoroughly documented:
- Physiotherapists will often have the best day-to-day news on motor impairments.
- OTs may help in the assessment of neglect and apraxias, and will start collecting information of the home environment and support.
- Speech and language therapists may report on progress with communication and swallowing.
- Nurses will know best about day-to-day functional performance.
- Problems emerging in functional tasks may prompt medial review (pain, breathlessness, dizziness, depression).

Any of these may collect information about pre-morbid abilities and home circumstances. In this case, demarcation between professions is not clear cut. Share information and avoid duplication if possible (if nothing else, it undermines the confidence of patients and carers to be asked the same information three or four times).

Moving on

What happens after the acute ward depends on how services are config-
ured in any one place:
- Some services combine acute and rehabilitation care.
- Some separate them out.
- Some combine stroke and generic rehabilitation.
- Others specialize.
- Some have well-developed home rehabilitation.

There is no clear cut-point when acute care becomes rehabilitation.
Involvement of rehabilitation therapists is beneficial at an early stage.
Continuity may be best served by keeping all stroke care in one place.

On the other hand, acute care and rehabilitation sometimes sit uncom-
fortably together. If you are worrying about drips and measuring blood
glucose, you are less likely to walk the patient to the toilet or make plans
for going home.

Size of the service, and availability of beds is also important. A large service
can justify separate wards better than a small one. And rehabilitation may of
necessity take place on an acute ward, while a place on a rehabilitation ward
is awaited.

There may be two important questions that need answering at this
point:
- Can the patient go home?
- Can the patient move to a rehabilitation ward?

Going home

We will discuss discharge planning, and options for home rehabilitation,
later. 'Can this patient go home?' must be asked at an early stage. For this
to succeed:
- The patient must be medically stable (i.e. neurologically stable, free
  from debilitating infection, severe metabolic disturbance, or
  cardiorespiratory problems such as hypotension, unstable cardiac
  rhythms, untreated heart or respiratory failure, acute coronary
  syndromes).
- Able to feed and maintain hydration adequately.
- As a minimum, be able to transfer to the commode by day and
  at night, alone or with a willing carer.
- Plans made for pressure area relief.
- Plans made for managing continence problems.
- Plans made for delivering medication.
- Plans made for continuing rehabilitation, if required, at home, in a day
  hospital or as an out-patient.

If 'returning home' means returning to a residential or nursing home, be
aware of the difference between them:
- A residential home provides 'board, lodging, and personal care'.
  Although criteria vary, they cannot as a rule cope with severely
  disabled or ill patients.
- Nursing homes have at least one registered nurse on duty all the time,
  and they can cope with much severer levels of disability. But they are

not hospitals. If and when to discharge is a matter for negotiation between the patient, the home, and your (team's) assessment of how well the setting can provide for any ongoing rehabilitation needs.

Transfer to a rehabilitation ward

Rehabilitation wards vary. Some may take patients early, and manage 'acute' problems such as dysphagia. Some provide very intensive rehabilitation. They may require patients to be:

- Fully alert.
- Cognitively able to follow instructions and retain ('carry over') what is learnt.
- Robust enough to take part in rehabilitation without tiring unduly.
- Free from major comorbidity.

Given the nature of the population, the system must also include wards that will take on as many problems as the patient presents. These may include cognitive impairment, multiple comorbidities and lack of stamina. However, a designated rehabilitation ward, which may be off the acute general hospital site, could reasonably expect a patient to be:

- Medically stable.
- Free from infectious diarrhoea (including *Clostridium difficile*—although MRSA colonization should not necessarily be a bar to management on a rehabilitation ward).
- Able to swallow safely, and maintain adequate nutrition.
- Not imminently awaiting tests or opinions, such as CT scans, necessitating an unpleasant ambulance journey back to the acute hospital, and possibly tying up a member of staff for a morning.
- There is no evidence to suggest that those with more severe stroke benefit less from active attempts at rehabilitation in specialized units (Box 3.1).

Box 3.1 Stroke unit care is beneficial to patients who have suffered a severe stroke

- 71 patients with severe stroke (selected by initial neurological features, the Orpington Prognostic Score) were randomized between a stroke unit and general ward management.
- Mortality was 21% (stroke unit) vs. 46% (general wards).
- Home discharge rate was 47% (stroke unit) vs. 21% (general ward).
- Median length of hospital stay was 43 days (stroke unit) vs. 59 days (general ward).

Stroke 1995; **26**: 2031–4

What do specialist services do differently?

Specialist services improve outcomes (Box 3.2). The exact reasons are uncertain, but some combination of (multiprofessional) expertise, thoroughness, continuity, and enthusiasm for managing stroke patients clearly makes a difference (Boxes 3.3 and 3.4).

Box 3.2 Improved outcomes with specialist stroke unit management

- Between the 1970s and 2000, 23 RCTs compared management in geographically defined stroke units with general medical wards.
- Stroke units varied greatly. Predominantly they were rehabilitation units, some were acute wards, others were mixed.
- RRs for stroke unit over general ward care were:
  - 0.80 (95%CI 0.60–1.0) for all cause mortality
  - 0.68 (95%CI 0.52–0.84) for combined death or dependency.
- There were no differences in benefits according to age, sex, stroke severity, type of medical department providing the service, timing of admission, or maximum duration of stay.
- Mean length of stay on the stroke units varied from 13 to 162 days, which was in some cases shorter, and others longer, than for the control group. Overall there was little difference.
- There was no clear benefit for dedicated stroke wards over mixed rehabilitation wards (odds ratio for death plus dependency 1.01, 95% CI 0.51–1.51).
- Characteristics of stroke units differing from general wards were co-ordinated multidisciplinary management, involvement of family in rehabilitation, specialization, and education of staff patients and carers (features you would expect on any good rehabilitation ward).
- Stroke outcomes are sensitive to differences in process, but the most important individual elements remain uncertain.

British Medical Journal 1997; **314**: 1151–9; *Cochrane Library* 2004; Issue 2.

Box 3.3 Possible explanations for better outcomes on stroke units

- Amount of remedial therapy.
- Therapy type or content.
- Aids, appliances, orthoses, and seating.
- Better identification of stroke-associated impairments and disabilities.
- Assessment and management of comorbidity.
- Prevention, identification, and management of complications.
- Continuity (nurses adopting therapy principles, routines, policies).
- Less competition for medical and nursing time.
- Improved motivation, morale, and psychological support.
- Increased self-directed therapy.
- Communication, education, and involvement of relatives.
- Realistic goal setting and prognostication.
- Discharge planning.
- Follow-up and outreach for late complications.

Box 3.4 How specialist services are different in practice

- An observational study, embedded in a RCT (Box 2.1) identified differences in care between a stroke unit and general wards receiving advice from stroke specialists.
- The stroke unit had guidelines for diagnosis, imaging, monitoring (BP, oxygen saturation, blood glucose, fluids and electrolytes, nutrition), and prevention of complications (positioning, swallow assessment, infections, venous thrombosis). Management was multidisciplinary, with early mobilization, individualized rehabilitation plans, and active patient participation.
- The general wards had a peripatetic specialist stroke team, who confirmed the diagnosis and made medical, therapy, and nursing plans, which were implemented by ward staff. The team reviewed patients, set goals, planned treatment and discharge, and liaised with relatives.
- Most aspects of care were comparable, and some differences quite small. However, stroke unit patients were:
  - more thoroughly assessed and monitored for neurological status;
  - more often given oxygen, paracetamol for pyrexia, anticoagulated for atrial fibrillation, screened for swallowing problems, fed early (oral, nasogastrically or PEG in first 7 days);
  - assessed earlier by OT and social worker;
  - more often given rehabilitation goals, including higher level tasks and carer needs;
  - given better secondary prevention;
  - given more information (as were carers).
- Stroke progression, chest and other infections, dehydration, pressure sores, injurious falls and other complications were less common on the stroke unit.
- Good outcomes were associated with measures to prevent aspiration, early feeding, and lack of stroke progression, chest infection, and dehydration, but not euglycaemia, or use of oxygen or antipyretics, in a multivariate analysis.
- Even after taking these into account, stroke unit management remained associated with better outcomes, suggesting that other undefined factors were also important.

Lancet 2001; **358**: 1586–92

Summary

1. During the first 2 weeks, some patients die, others recover completely. Some are left with minor disability, with the prospect of rapid rehabilitation and discharge home. Others remain medically and neurologically unstable, and if they survive, have major disability and may need prolonged rehabilitation.
2. If swallowing is unsafe 2 days after the stroke, consider passing a nasogastric tube. If the problem persists beyond 2 weeks, consider a gastrostomy (remembering these take few days to organize). Involve a speech and language therapist.
3. Medical complications and neurological deterioration should prompt thorough medical review, to ascertain the diagnosis and institute appropriate management.
4. Bladder and bowel management in the acute phase centres around excluding easily reversible causes, and then adequate containment until the patient is well enough to consider other options.
5. Make early referrals to physiotherapy and OTs.
6. Case notes should be thorough and systematic, recording information from both the medical and functional perspectives. Multidisciplinary team communication should be regular, and well documented.
7. When medically stable and able to maintain nutrition, the patient may move on to either home rehabilitation, or a rehabilitation ward, depending on local services.

Subarachnoid haemorrhage

SAH may initially look like a stroke, but behaves differently. Specialist management is the province of the neurosurgeon, but general and stroke physicians need some grounding in its diagnosis and management.

Incidence is about one-tenth that of other strokes: 10–15 per 100 000 per year. Half present between ages 40 and 55. A third occur during sleep, a third during strenuous activity or lifting, and a third during other daytime activities.

What it is

The intracranial vessels lie in the subarachnoid space giving off branches to the brain. Primary SAH occurs when a blood vessel ruptures and blood enters the subarachnoid space. Secondary SAH is an extension from a primary intracerebral haemorrhage, or from trauma.

Causes of primary SAH include:
- Ruptured arterial aneurysms (85% of cases, excluding trauma).
- Perimesencephalic SAH (around the brainstem, of uncertain origin, probably venous, 10%).
- Ruptured arteriovenous malformation.
- Rarer causes:
  - bleeding disorders (including thrombocytopenia, leukaemias)
  - anticoagulant therapy
  - bleeding from tumours
  - mycotic aneurysms from endocarditis
  - vertebral arterial dissection
  - cocaine abuse
  - vasculitis.

Blood in the subarachnoid space raises intracranial pressure, irritates the meninges, and causes vasospasm. This produces headache, neck stiffness, risk of coning, and secondary ischaemic brain damage.

Clinical presentation

- Headache, unusually severe, with abrupt (split second) onset, often described as 'being hit on the back of the head' or an explosion. This may be preceded (in 25%) by a few milder attacks of headache or 'warning leaks'.
- Loss of consciousness may follow the headache (in 50%, but it may be brief). Half never wake up. Others are drowsy but not unconscious. Onset may be with a fit (10%).
- You cannot rule out SAH clinically in a patient with sudden onset headache lasting over 2 h, even if there are no other symptoms or signs. Twenty-five per cent of sudden onset headaches are due to SAH, half this if there are no other features. There is no alternative to getting a CT scan.
- Headache onset may be slower (minutes) in perimesencephalic SAH. Loss of consciousness and focal neurology do not occur.
- Some are confused and irritable (delirious), some vomit at onset, some develop photophobia.
- Signs of meningism develop 3–12 h after onset—neck stiffness and Kernig's sign (resistance to knee extension with the hip flexed).
- Some patients also develop early focal neurological signs such as hemiplegia or cranial nerve palsies due to pressure from blood clot or aneurysm, or raised intracranial pressure.
- Hypertension occurs in 50% (some pre-existing, most reactive to the raised intracranial pressure).
- Pyrexia, not due to infection, is common, and may persist for several days. It is associated with poorer outcomes. Half of pyrexial patients have pneumonia, however.
- Examination of the optic fundus may show papilloedema, subhyaloid haemorrhage (in 20%), or vitreous haemorrhage.
- Tendon reflexes may be depressed and plantar responses upgoing.
- An enlarging aneurysm can compress cranial nerves, which may precede rupture (by hours to days):
  - internal carotid or anterior communicating artery (optic nerve or chiasm—retro-orbital pain and unilateral visual loss);
  - internal carotid: cavernous sinus wall
    - oculomotor (III) nerve—palsy (±Horners)
    - trochlear (IV) nerve—palsy
    - ophthalmic division of the facial (V) nerve—pain
    - abducens (VI) nerve—palsy.
  - posterior communicating or basilar artery—retro-orbital pain, and oculomotor (III) palsy;
  - IIIrd and VIth nerve palsy can also indicate tentorial herniation.

Diagnosis

- CT head scan. Confirms the diagnosis in 95% of cases, if the scan is done within 48 h. Sensitivity is only 50% after a week's delay.
- When the scan is positive, the blood may be:
  - widespread in the basal cisterns and interhemispheric fissure;
  - intraventricular (a fluid level in the posterior part of the lateral ventricle);
  - localized to the site of the ruptured aneurysm, such as the Sylvian fissure from the middle cerebral artery, or interhemispheric fissure due to ruptured anterior communicating artery;
  - free blood over the cortical sulci;
  - perimesencephalic haemorrhage (seen in 10%, not usually associated with aneurysms)—blood is around the mid-brain in the interpeduncular fossa, with no extension to the brain or ventricular systems;
  - in addition there may be:
    - hydrocephalus
    - intracerebral haemorrhage
    - tumours
    - ateriovenous malformations.
- Lumbar puncture. If the history is suggestive, *and CT scan is negative*, do a lumbar puncture:
  - to make the diagnosis and rule out meningitis, provided more than 6 h has elapsed from the onset of the headache;
  - do not do a lumbar puncture if the patient has unreversed anticoagulation (INR >1.5) or thrombocytopenia (platelets $<50 \times 10^9$/l), or if a supratentorial mass lesion has not been excluded;
  - negative in 10–15% of SAH;
  - red blood cells are present for 2–3 days after SAH. They can also contaminate CSF after a traumatic tap. Six hours after SAH, however, the CSF becomes yellow (xanthochromia), and this can be detected spectrophotometrically. There is also a slightly raised protein and monocytosis.
  - xanthochromia persists for 2 weeks, so can be used to investigate patients who present late after onset of headache;
- Angiography shows an aneurysm in 85%. Ten per cent have more than one aneurysm. Choice of MRA (90% sensitive), CTA, or conventional catheter angiography depends on local availability and expertise.

'Grading' of subarachnoid haemorrhages

The World Federation of Neurological Surgery grades SAHs according to the presenting features (Table 4.1), which guides intervention and prognosis.

Remember that you must diagnose the cause of depressed consciousness. Acute hydrocephalus (progressive drowsiness over first few hours), and comorbid metabolic disorders, are treatable.

There are other prognostic grading systems, so be careful about which one is being referred to.

Table 4.1 World Federation of Neurological Surgery grades for SAH

Grade	GCS	Focal deficits
I	15	Absent
II	13–14	Absent
III	13–14	Present
IV	7–12	Present or absent
V	3–6	Present or absent

Initial management of subarachnoid haemorrhage

- Manage on a high-dependency, critical care or neurosurgical ward.
- Bed rest until the aneurysm is clipped or coiled.
- Monitor the Glasgow Coma Scale. Deterioration can mean ischaemia, rebleeding, hydrocephalus, or systemic medical complications.
- Pass a nasogastric tube unless swallowing safely.
- Give paracetamol (1 g qds by mouth or per rectum) or codeine (30–60 mg qds by mouth, nasogastric tube or SC) for headache. Avoid sedative drugs.
- Give a stool softener (sodium docusate 200 mg bd).
- Give IV saline 3 l/day (in addition to enteral intake, giving a total intake up to 6 l/day), to prevent hypovolaemia and hyponatraemia due to 'cerebral salt wasting'.
- Monitor fluid balance, measure urea and electrolytes daily.
- Give nimodipine 60 mg every 4 h by mouth or nasogastric tube for 21 days, so long as systolic BP is more than 100 mmHg (reduces risk of delayed cerebral ischaemia and poor outcomes—Box 4.1).
- Apart from oral nimodipine do not generally try to lower BP. Any reduction in rebleeding is offset by increased risk of infarction. Previous antihypertensive drugs can be continued if the BP is not too low (<140 mmHg systolic).
- Liaise early with a neurosurgeon (and/or neuroradiologists) about the strategy for imaging and possible operative intervention. The patient will usually need to be transferred to a neurosurgical centre.
- If there is an associated intraparenchymal haematoma (30% of cases), and progressive decrease in level of consciousness (over the first 2 days) immediate surgical evacuation should be considered. This may prevent herniation, and minimize the volume of damaged brain.
- Progressive reduction in level of consciousness (possibly with sluggish pupillary responses to light and downward deviation of the eyes), over a few hours, may be due to acute hydrocephalus. Confirm with CT head scan, and refer to a neurosurgeon.

Box 4.1 Trial of nimodipine in subarachnoid haemorrhage

- 554 patients with proven SAH, admitted within 96 h, were randomized to 21 days of oral (or nasogastric) nimodipine 60 mg 4 hourly or placebo.
- Patients who had SAH producing coma within the week prior to the index event were excluded, otherwise exclusion criteria were minimal.
- 77% of patients had an aneurysm at angiography.
- RRs on treatment were:
  - 0.66 (95% CI 0.50–0.87) for cerebral infarction (33% vs. 22%);
  - 0.60 (95% CI 0.45–0.80) for death or severe disability (33% vs. 20%);
  - 0.71 (95% CI 0.50–1.01) for death (22% vs. 15%);
  - 0.65 (95% CI 0.41–1.05) for rebleeding (9% vs. 4%).
- Effect of treatment was independent of prognostic factors (including loss of consciousness at onset, age, time to entry, focal neurological signs, and CT and angiographic findings).
- Results were supported in a subsequent meta-analysis, but not where nimodipine was given IV.

British Medical Journal 1989; **298**: 636–42

Selection for imaging and surgery

- Patients in 'good grades' (conscious and without focal neurological signs), and who would be willing to have surgery, should have early angiography.
- If the first angiogram is negative it should be repeated a few days later, unless the bleeding pattern on CT is perimesencephalic.
- Those with a surgically amenable aneurysm that has bled will usually have this clipped. Aneurysm surgery is performed within 3 days of initial bleed or after 12 days.
- Early surgery may prevent re-bleeds, and reduce delayed ischaemia, but overall there are no clear differences in outcomes between early and late surgery.
- Coiling (endovascularly, performed by interventional neuroradiologists) is an increasingly popular alternative to surgery (Box 4.2).

Box 4.2 Endovascular coiling or neurosurgical clipping for ruptured aneurysms (International Subarachnoid Aneurysm Trial—ISAT)

- 2143 patients with ruptured intracranial aneurysms randomized to neurosurgical clipping or endovascular coiling (when the aneurysm was technically suitable for either treatment—22% of patients presenting).
- Mean age was 52 years, range 18–87, 88% were WFNS grade 1 or 2. Most were small anterior circulation aneurysms. (Coiling is preferred anyway for posterior circulation aneurysms because of surgical risk, and surgery is generally preferred for middle cerebral artery aneurysms.)
- About 5% of patients allocated to coiling required neurosurgery.
- RRs for coiling compared with surgery, at 12 months, were:
  - 0.88 (95% CI 0.73–1.06) for deaths (8% vs. 10%);
  - 0.77 (95% CI 0.66–0.91) for death or dependency (24% vs. 31%).
- Grade, age, amount of blood, and lumen size had no effect on RRs.
- Rebleeding risk up to 1 year was 22 vs. 21. After 1 year rebleeding risk was 2 in 1276 patient-years for coiling, and 0 in 1081 patient-years for surgery. A higher risk of bleeding postcoiling was off-set by a greater delay before neurosurgery, during which some pre-procedure re-bleeds occurred.
- In technically suitable aneurysms, treated in centres with sufficient expertise, endovascular coiling improves the chances of independent survival.

Lancet 2002; **360**: 1267–74

Non-operative management

- In perimesencephalic SAH, angiography is advised, but usually there is no aneurysm. Treat the headache and mobilize.
- In (proven or presumed) aneurysmal SAH:
  - conservative management is reserved for patients too ill to withstand surgery (WFNS grades 3–5), with severe comorbidity, or where there are particular technical operative risks—the neurosurgeon (and anaesthetist) should be the ones to decide this;
  - consider coiling where fitness for open surgery is in doubt;
  - otherwise, bed rest for 3 weeks;
  - treat headache (paracetamol, codeine), give stool softeners (sodium docusate 200 mg bd);
  - general care of the unconscious or very ill patient—pressure areas, nutrition, anti-embolism stockings;
  - later investigation and surgery may be possible for initially poor grade patients who subsequently improve;
  - mortality is very high.

Neurological complications

Neurological complications of SAH are listed in Table 4.2.
There are two types of hydrocephalus:

- Early obstructive hydrocephalus due to blood clots in the ventricular system. Occurs within 7 days of SAH. Ventriculostomy can be life saving, but increases the risk of re-bleeding (reduced counter pressure).
- Later communicating hydrocephalus. May be due to blood within the basal cisterns or obstruction of the arachnoid villi. Seen in 10–20% over following weeks and months. This needs ventriculoperitoneal shunting.
- Suspect it in any patient with SAH who develops one or more of:
  - headache
  - gradual deterioration of consciousness
  - impairment of cognitive function
  - incontinence
  - gait ataxia.

Non-neurological complications of subarachnoid haemorrhage

- Acute MI. Transient ECG changes, and histological subendocardial infarction, are very common.
- Cardiac arrhythmias, including ventricular tachycardia. Rarely needs treatment.
- Acute pulmonary oedema. Rapid onset, usually in severe SAH. Treat with oxygen, diuretics, or ventilation.
- Reactive hypertension.
- Delirium due to drugs, alcohol or benzodiazepine withdrawal, or medical complications.
- Gastric ulcer (stress ulcer) with or without bleeding.
- Hyponatraemia and reduced plasma volume:
  - develops 2nd–10th day
  - caused by natriuresis (cerebral salt wasting), not SIADH
  - 10% have serum sodium concentration less than 125 mmol/l
  - severe hyponatraemia causes drowsiness, irritability, confusion, and seizures
  - 30% lose more than 10% of plasma volume—reduced plasma volume may reduce cerebral perfusion, and contribute to delayed ischaemia
  - anticipate the problem by giving saline, or dextrose saline
  - strict fluid balance monitoring. Insert a urinary catheter if need be, and may need to monitor central venous pressure. Give albumin if crystalloid is insufficient to maintain filling pressure
  - if using more than isotonic saline in severe hyponatraemia beware over-rapid (>0.5 mmol/l per hour) correction, which can lead to central pontine myelinolysis
  - add fludrocortisone 100–300 μg/day if sodium does not increase.

Table 4.2 Neurological complications of SAH

Complication	Features	Action
Rebleeding	Sudden worsening of headache with or without loss of consciousness. 20% on the first day, 40% in the first month (without intervention). On-going risk without surgery is high. 1/3 have initial respiratory arrest, of whom half recover spontaneous respiration within 24 h. 50% mortality.	Repeat CT scan (shows rebleed in 80%). Exclude other causes of decreased level of consciousness (found in 1/3). Ventilation is justified for respiratory arrest. Consider emergency surgery for aneurysm clipping.
Cerebral ischaemia (vasospasm)	About 25% incidence, usually between days 4–12, peaking at days 6–8, resolving over 2–4 weeks. 25% get focal deficits, 25% drowsiness, 50% both. 25% die. 10% of survivors severely disabled.	Urgent 'triple H'—hypervolaemia, haemodilution, hypertension. Transfer to HDU/ITU. Arterial line, central venous pressure monitoring. Volume expand with albumin (500 ml 5%). Stop nimodipine. Increase BP 20–40 mmHg with inotropes. Repeat CT.
Hydrocephalus	20% of unoperated patients. Half are initially alert. By time of diagnosis 70–90% drowsy, more as time goes by. May have small pupils, headache, or confusion.	Discuss with neurosurgeon. If alert or not too drowsy wait and see for 24 h. Half improve, but may fluctuate. Consider serial LP over 10 days if no obstruction, brain shift, haematoma or intraventricular haemorrhage on CT (remove 20 ml each time, target closing pressure 15 cmH$_2$O). Otherwise external drainage, at risk of increased rebleeding and infection.
Expanding haematoma	Progressive drowsiness over first few days.	Consider urgent surgical evacuation. Otherwise supportive only.
Epilepsy	10% within a month, mostly early.	Terminate with IV lorazepam, diazepam, or phenytoin. IV phenytoin maintenance.

Summary

1. Definitive SAH management is specialized, and involves neurosurgeons and neuroradiologists. Consult urgently with a neurosurgeon.
2. The initial priority is making the diagnosis. All patients with sudden onset persisting headache need a CT head scan, and lumbar puncture (after 6 h) if this is not diagnostic.
3. Oral (or nasogastric) nimodipine improves outcomes.
4. Pain control, fluid and electrolyte management, and complications need special attention. Manage in a high-dependency ward. Avoid sedative drugs.
5. Watch for deterioration (re-bleeding, hydrocephalus, ischaemia, fitting).
6. Patients in 'good grades' (initially alert) require angiography and work-up for clipping or coiling of the aneurysm.
7. Patients with poor prognosis or not fit for surgery may subsequently recover enough to allow intervention.

Chapter 5

Neuroimaging in stroke

Introduction

- Options for brain imaging include CT and MRI.
- In addition, intracranial haemorrhage (especially SAH), and work-up for carotid endarterectomy, may require vascular imaging (conventional angiography, MR angiography or contrast CT angiography).
- Suspected arterial dissection will require imaging (MRI/MRA, CTA, duplex scanning, or conventional angiography).

This chapter concentrates on the basics of brain imaging. It does not aim to make you into a neuroradiologist. It will help you understand the role of imaging and techniques employed, as an aid to intelligent ordering and interpretation of results.

By convention, the left side of the brain anatomically appears on the right side of the scan (the image is seen as if looked at from the feet upwards, with the patient on his or her back).

Computed tomography

CT scanning of the brain is the best imaging technique for initial investigation of acute stroke.

A standard CT scan of the brain consists of axial images through the whole brain. It is made by moving an X-ray beam synchronously with detectors across a slice of the brain. The X-rays transmitted through an element, or pixel, of the slice (<1mm) are processed by a computer, which gives a numerical value to its density. The range of the densities are measured as Hounsfield numbers, with values of −1000, 0, and +1000 for air, water, and bone, respectively. Difference in X-ray attenuation make it possible to differentiate normal and infarcted tissue, clotted or extravasated blood, tumour, or oedema.

In selected situations, IV injection of a non-ionic iodinated contrast agent is given to demonstrate breakdown of the blood–brain barrier or abnormal vessels, or to get a CT angiogram.

Advantages and disadvantages of computed tomography brain scanning

Advantages
- Widely available and non-invasive.
- Fast.
- Good sensitivity for many neurological conditions, including:
  - cerebral infarction
  - intracranial bleeding:
    - primary and secondary intracerebral haemorrhage
    - SAH
    - subdural haematoma
    - extradural haematoma
  - brain tumours
  - cerebral abscess
  - mid-line shift
  - hydrocephalus
  - brain atrophy
  - cerebral trauma.

Disadvantages
- Relatively heavy radiation dose (in context, more a theoretical than practical problem, unless the patient is pregnant).
- Early (<6–8 h) infarction may not be visible.
- Cannot show lesions involving brainstem or other parts of the brain within the posterior fossa very clearly.
- Insensitive to small lesions (<1 cm).
- May miss some lesions such as:
  - isodense subdural haematoma
  - low attenuation lesions near the skull
  - multiple sclerosis plaques
  - haemorrhage after 2 weeks.

Computed tomography scanning and intracranial haemorrhages

- Acute haemorrhage is visible on CT scan immediately. Recent blood clot, bleeding within the brain parenchyma (Figure 5.1), ventricular system, subarachnoid space (Figures 5.2 and 5.3), subdural or extradural spaces appear as hyperdensity, i.e. whiter than the brain parenchyma. This allows positive diagnosis of haemorrhagic stroke, and its exclusion. Chronic subdural haemorrhage is seen as an area of low attenuation compressing the brain from outside (Figure 5.4).
- The area of the increased density can be of any size or shape in patients with intracerebral bleeding, and often is surrounded by an area of low attenuation (darker) due to oedema, ischaemia, or clot retraction (Figure 5.1).
- When the haemorrhage is large, it may cause mid-line shift.
- Large supratentorial haematomas may cause herniation of the temporal lobe through the tentorial hiatus and compression of the brainstem or of the ipsilateral parasagittal cortex under the falx, compressing the ipsilateral lateral ventricle.
- Primary or secondary intracerebral bleeds may be associated with intraventricular bleeding (indicating poor prognosis).

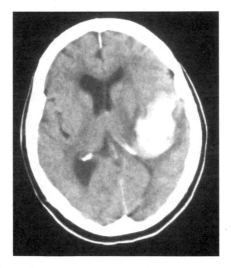

Fig. 5.1 Primary intracerebral haemorrhage. CT head. There is a large intra-cerebral haemorrhage in the left parieto-temporal lobe causing compression of the left lateral ventricle and minimal midline shift.

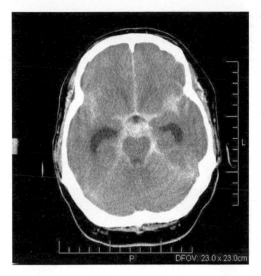

Fig. 5.2 Sub-arachnoid haemorrhage. CT head. Blood around the base of the brain secondary to a ruptured basilar aneurysm, and acute hydrocephalus.

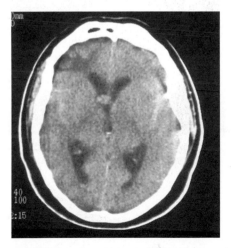

Fig. 5.3 Sub-arachnoid haemorrhage with intraventricular extension and acute hydrocephalus. CT head. There is blood in the subarachnoid space, particularly in the left sylvian fissure. There is extensive oedema, and an infarct in the right frontal lobe.

- Hypertensive bleeds tend to be in the basal ganglia, pons, or cerebellum.
- Lobar bleeds tend to occur from aneurysms, arteriovenous malformations, clotting disorders, or amyloid angiopathy.
- Within a few days to a few weeks, the haematoma becomes isodense and subsequently hypodense (dark). Similar CT scan changes occur with other types of intracranial bleeding, including subdural haematoma (Figure 5.4).
- IV contrast may help to diagnose haemorrhages into tumours that otherwise may be missed.
- After about a week, IV contrast may show a ring enhancement around the haematoma, which can mimic cerebral tumours or abscesses.

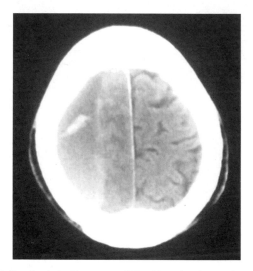

Fig. 5.4 Chronic sub-dural haematoma. CT head. Large low-density right chronic sub-dural haematoma with some acute bleeding into it.

Computed tomography scanning for cerebral infarction

- In the first 24 h, CT scan may be normal in patients with cerebral infarction, particularly those with small lesions. Up to 40% of stroke patients may never have a visible lesion.
- Sometimes ischaemic changes can be seen as early as 1 h after stroke onset, but are seen more reliably after 3–6 h. Early signs of ischaemia include:
  - occluded vessel—hyperdense middle cerebral (or other) artery, due to a clot in the artery (seen in 20–40%, but less reliable in elderly people);
  - loss of grey–white matter differentiation, particularly loss of visualization of the insular ribbon;
  - effacement of overlying cortical sulci (mass effect due to oedema);
  - loss of outline of the lentiform nucleus of the basal ganglia;
  - low density in the cortex and subcortical white matter.
- A fully evolved cerebral infarction is seen as an area of low attenuation, which is due to increased water content of the cells (Figures 5.5–5.8, pp. 105–6).
  If the infarction is extensive, the brain swelling and oedema may occur within the first 24 h causing mid-line shift.
- Haemorrhagic transformation may occur and will be shown as increased density at the centre of the infarction:
  - a frank haematoma
  - a diffuse speckled petechial pattern.
- During the second week the infarction increases in density and may become isodense, making the infarcted area similar to the surrounding brain.
- Brainstem and cerebellar infarctions may be visible (Figure 5.6) but if they are small, can be difficult to visualize due to bone artefacts.
- Old infarctions are seen as well-demarcated hypodense lesions (holes) with similar density to that of the CSF.

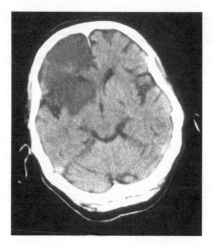

Fig. 5.5 Middle cerebral artery territory infarct. CT head. There is a large low attenuation area in the right fronto-parietal region with compression of the lateral ventricle but no midline displacement.

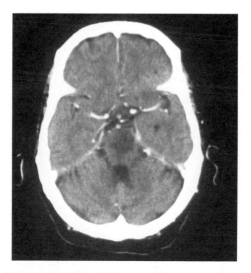

Fig. 5.6 Brainstem infarct. CT head with contrast. There is a non-enhancing low attenuation area in the left side of the pons and midbrain. The middle cerebral and basilar arteries can be clearly seen.

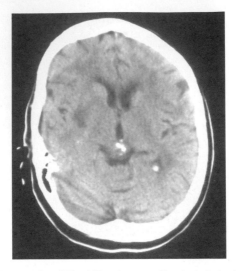

Fig. 5.7 Lacunar infarct. CT head. There is an area of low density in the right basal ganglia.

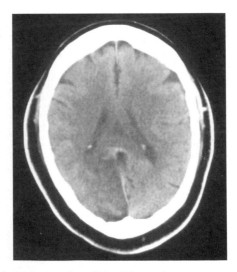

Fig. 5.8 Occipital cortex infarct. CT head. There is a low attenuation area in the right occipital region. The anatomical distribution is that of the right posterior cerebral artery.

Magnetic resonance imaging

MRI detects the presence, and mobility, of hydrogen atoms, and therefore water. T1 weighted images show brain structure. T2 weighted images show areas with high water content as white (e.g. CSF, infarction, oedema).

Advantages

- Radiation-free.
- The pictures are technically superior.
- More sensitive for cerebral infarction, especially in the posterior fossa and lacunar infarction.
- MR angiography can be performed at the same time (without the need for contrast).
- Diffusion-weighted images are very sensitive to early infarction (30 min after onset).
- Perfusion-weighted images (with contrast) give an indication of cerebral perfusion, and can be compared with diffusion-weighted images to reveal areas of mismatch (poor perfusion, but not yet infarcted), which represents the potentially salvageable penumbra.
- MR venography is investigation of choice for venous sinus thrombosis.
- Can detect vasculitis.

Disadvantages

- Relatively slow and noisy, with poorer access for monitoring. Ten per cent of patients cannot be examined due to claustrophobia. Scan times are getting much quicker, however.
- Possibly less able to detect early haemorrhage (but more sensitive after about 24 h).
- Intracranial metal aneurysm clips, pacemakers, intraocular metallic foreign bodies, cochlear implants and programmable hydrocephalus shunts are contraindications to cranial MRI scanning. Other metal prostheses should be notified in advance to the scanning department.

Infarction on magnetic resonance imaging

- Early signs are a loss of the normal flow void in the affected artery (immediate), bright images on diffusion weighting (Figure 5.9), swelling on T1, and intense bright signal on T2 (6 h), which remains bright for 1–2 weeks (Figures 1.3e, 5.10 and 5.11).
- After this lesions may become isointense with normal brain.
- After several weeks infarcts look like CSF (dark T1, bright T2).

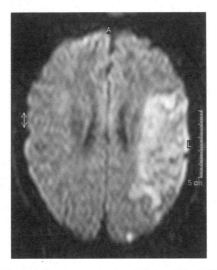

Fig. 5.9 Middle cerebral artery territory infarct. Diffusion-weighted MRI showing infarction in the left fronto-parietal lobe.

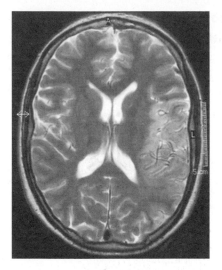

Fig. 5.10 Middle cerebral artery territory infarct. T2-weighted MRI showing infarction in the left fronto-parietal lobe.

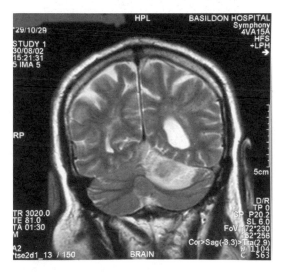

Fig. 5.11 Cerebellar infarct. T2-weighted MRI, coronal section, showing infarction in the left cerebellar hemisphere.

Haemorrhage on magnetic resonance imaging

- MRI signals vary according to the age of the haemorrhage, but this should not be a problem in experienced hands, and with special MR sequences (T2* and echo gradient).
- Early appearances may be confused with infarction. There may be a bright core, with a dark rim of deoxyhaemoglobin, and bright surrounding oedema.
- After about 24 h blood becomes dark on T1 and T2 images.
- Over the next week the T1 image becomes bright again as methaemoglobin forms.
- After a week the T2 image becomes bright as well.
- After several weeks a dark ring (haemosiderin) forms around the haemorrhage on T2 images, which persists (useful in diagnosing a late presentation).

Summary

1. CT scan of the head is the initial investigation of choice. It should be performed urgently if bleeding, SAH, tumour, or abscess is suspected, if there is unexplained coma, or thrombolysis is being considered. Otherwise it should be performed within 24 h of onset. It can distinguish infarcts from bleeds, and identify most non-vascular pathologies mimicking stroke.

2. CT scan may not detect early infarction, but is very sensitive for detecting bleeds.

3. MRI is especially useful in examining the posterior fossa, and is more sensitive than CT in identifying lacunar infarcts. Diffusion-weighted images have excellent sensitivity very early after infarction.

4. Discuss urgent, contentious, difficult, or unusual requests with the radiologist.

Chapter 6

Making difficult decisions

Consent

Most healthcare interventions require consent. Merely touching someone without their permission may constitute 'battery'. Doing anything which might (to the legal mind) constitute an injury, may be an assault. Health professionals are unused to thinking like this, but some patients, lawyers, and governments do.

The key points are:

- You must get consent before you examine, investigate, treat, or otherwise care for a competent adult patient.
- Consent may be *explicit* (permission asked and granted), or *implied* (the patient comes to you voluntarily, asks for help, co-operates, and does not object to what you are proposing or doing, e.g. holding his or her arm out so you can take blood).
- Explicit consent can be *written*, or *verbal*, and both are equally valid (although the latter is harder to prove).
- An adult is anyone over the age of 18 years. In the UK, between ages 16 and 18, and for younger children who can understand what is involved (so-called 'Gillick-competent' minors), matters are more complicated. The patient can give his or her own consent, as can a parent, but he or she cannot withhold consent (for arcane legal reasons). Otherwise, a parent must consent, except in an emergency.
- Always assume an adult is competent (or '*has capacity*') to give or withhold consent unless you can demonstrate otherwise.
- Patients may be competent to make some decisions, but not others, and their ability to consent may vary with time. Patients may change their mind about consenting (or not consenting).
- A decision that you find surprising, or with which you disagree, does not prove that the patient does not have capacity. Competent adults may refuse any treatment, even if it would clearly benefit their health, unless it is treatment of a mental illness and they are detained under the Mental Health Act.
- Consent must be 'informed'—otherwise it is invalid. This means patients need sufficient information to be able to come to a decision, such as benefits and risks, and possible alternative treatments.
- Consent must also be voluntary—not under any duress from relatives, friends, or staff.
- In England, no one can give consent on behalf of an adult who does not have capacity to consent. They may be treated if it is in their 'best interests'. Elsewhere (e.g. Scotland) a representative may have been legally appointed who has authority to take decisions for an incapacitated patient.

Capacity

Assessing capacity is asking whether someone can understand and weigh up information necessary to make a decision. To have capacity to consent a patient must:

- Understand the nature, purpose, and effects of the treatment.
- Understand any adverse effects, any alternative treatments, and the consequences of refusal.
- Be able to take in, retain, believe, and weigh up the information to make a judgement.
- Communicate a decision.
- Do so free from undue pressure.

Understanding need only be in broad terms. This is fortunate, as you might imagine that on these criteria a large proportion of your patients cannot give their own consent. Patients may be able to consent to some things, but not others.

How to make decisions

Classically four factors are involved:
- Beneficence, or doing good ('benefits').
- Non-maleficence, or avoiding harm ('burdens or risks').
- Autonomy.
- Justice, or equity.

The first two define whether an intervention is *effective* or not—is it technically feasible? Unless the likely good from a procedure outweighs the likely harm, or at least justifies it, it is not effective. Good and harm is judged in terms of effect on length of life, curing diseases, reducing symptoms or increasing abilities, avoiding complications and side-effects, and the short-term unpleasantness or debility associated with the procedure.

If a procedure is ineffective, or is highly unlikely to have its desired effect, it is said to be *futile*. In these cases consent is not generally an issue, as futile interventions should not be offered to patients. There may still be a need for, or an obligation to give, an explanation of why potential treatments are not being offered.

Assuming that there is a reasonable prospect of an intervention doing more good than harm, next consider *autonomy*. This is essentially the same as asking consent.

How you proceed depends on whether the patient has capacity to decide or not. Autonomy does not dictate that a futile procedure should be undertaken, even if the patient wants it, but otherwise the autonomy of competent patients must be respected. They can exercise it by refusing a treatment that might be effective. The only way of finding out what a patient wants is to ask them.

If a patient can give you the information you need, do not ask relatives or friends first. It is technically a breach of *confidentiality* to discuss things without the patient's permission, and their opinions may not accurately reflect those of the patient. If a patient does not have capacity, then we can still respect autonomy by trying to find out what they would have wanted (see below).

Equity and justice refer to two things:
- *Non-discrimination*; on the basis of things that should have no influence on decision making (sex, race, religion, political views, disability, age).
- *Rationing*, or fair shares; available resources must be used to maximize the good done overall to the greatest number of people. This is really the responsibility of politicians, and health administrators. It can make life difficult for doctors, because the clinical ethic demands that we do our best for the patient in front of us, ideally without taking account of resource issues. As a general rule use common sense.

Best interest

The idea of 'best interest' applies where a patient does not have capacity to give or withhold consent. In the UK, a treatment may be legally given, despite lack of consent, if it is in the patient's best interest.

The technical issue of effectiveness still holds—the benefits of treatment must outweigh the burdens. There are several formulations of this from published documents, that are useful when discussing the issues with involved parties (staff, relatives):

- Is the proposed treatment likely to lead to a length and quality of life that the patient would have found acceptable?
- Does the treatment make possible a decent life in which a patient can reasonably be thought to have a continued interest?

Both of these introduce ideas beyond the likely clinical outcome (length and quality of life). They include a need to respect the wishes of the patient. There are several levels of information:

- An *advanced directive*, or living will, may legally define in some detail what the patient would or would not have wanted done. Unfortunately very few people have made these (have you?—see http://www.tht.org.uk/publications/livingwill.htm). There will often be some doubt as to whether the exact circumstances intended by the patient actually apply.

- A *proxy judgement*: someone may be able to tell you what the patient would have said, because they had discussed the issues previously. The degree of uncertainty mounts when the exact circumstances have not been discussed, but opinions may still be known in general terms. This often comes down to asking 'knowing the person as you do, what do you think they would have wanted?'—which is a pretty rough and ready assessment of opinion.

- A *substitute judgement*: this asks what the informant (relative, friend, or staff member) would want in this situation. This may be useful when someone is of a particular religious faith, where general principles are well known. Staff making this judgement are essentially saying 'as a fellow human being what would I have wanted?'. This has some validity, but opinions do vary widely.

Be careful, as research has shown that some people with a condition view it as less bad than do staff members, relatives, or members of the general population (who are the most averse to descriptions of severe disability). The majority of the population, however, when asked, rate living with a severe stroke as bad as death or worse than death. A minority disagree.

Avoid giving the impression that you are asking family members to make life or death decisions. Legally these decisions have no validity (in England), and it is unfair to burden families with further distress and possible guilt, when they are having to cope with severe illness in a close relative. You are only asking what the patient would have wanted were they able to give their opinion.

All this requires some knowledge about:

- The condition.
- Its natural history.

- The effectiveness of treatment.
- What the patient would have wanted you to do.

There is usually uncertainty about all of these, which makes life difficult, and good judgement important. When the ethical framework is properly applied it is quite simple, and many nurses and junior doctors will have the necessary knowledge and skills. However, these discussions should usually involve the most senior doctor available. You should always be able to expect support, both in making decisions, and discussing them, or their consequences, if you need to.

Ultimate responsibility for deciding on best interest, and formally declaring it to be so, rests with the consultant in charge of the case. Senior staff may want support by discussing cases with colleagues, or asking second opinions.

Recently, there have been efforts to formalize the definition of best interest (Box 6.1).

Box 6.1. Proposed criteria for defining best interests in England and Wales

- Respect the patient's past and present views if possible.
- Encourage participation in the decision and care.
- Seek the opinion of family members, or others, whom it is appropriate and practical to consult.
- Use the least restrictive alternative option.
- Do not compromise patient safety (e.g. on the basis of observed behaviours or past experience).
- There is a general authority to *act reasonably* on behalf of someone without capacity.

Lord Chancellor's Department (2002).
http://www.lcd.gov.uk/menincap/ch3.htm#Anchor-Best

Managing decision making

We must make decisions well, be seen to make them well, and 'carry' staff and families with the process. The ideal is to reach consensus, and agreement. This is often possible, by explaining the process behind decision making, and showing that the health professional is not arbitrarily 'playing God'.

Sometimes, strong convictions and emotions raise barriers to what rational thought dictates. We must be sensitive to these—acknowledge them, show you understand them, take them into account or accept them. Remember, however, that acting against the 'best interest' of someone who cannot speak for themselves is an assault, and is technically illegal. Common sense must prevail. A 'cosmetic' drip may help a relative come to terms with the impending death of a family member. Avoid being dogmatic, but you must always be ready and able to justify what you have done after the event.

Sometimes, uncertainty in decision making means we must prevaricate. A holding operation for a few days (or weeks), such as IV hydration, while we see which way things are turning out, is perfectly acceptable if a decision can be postponed. We are gathering more information on which to base a final judgement.

Applying this to stroke care

Capacity to consent

The main problems are:
- coma;
- dysphasia;
- cognitive impairment due to stroke;
- comorbid dementia, learning disabilities, or delirium;
- other communication problems such as deafness;
- language barriers in non-English speakers—although the decisions are sufficiently important to justify getting a translator if no family member is bilingual and willing to help.

Medical interventions without consent in conditions that may only be temporary, should strictly be limited to those required to preserve life and immediate health. In practice, this rarely applies to stroke:
- We may not know how reversible the condition will be, e.g. cognitive impairment or dysphasia.
- Or how quickly it might reverse.
- Sometimes, if you are going to treat something at all, you need to treat quickly—such as antibiotics or rehydration.

As a general rule, if someone has presented to hospital, it is reasonable to give nursing and medical care (i.e. anything short of operative procedures), as you think is best practice and in their best interests, unless or until someone objects. At that point you can reassess more formally:
- Formally consider someone's capacity to consent.
- The nature of the objection.
- The likely alternatives.
- The status of the person objecting—clearly the views of the patient, a spouse or (adult) child have more weight than those of the next-door neighbour.
- Whether someone else has relevant information or views which must be sought prior to making a decision.
- What best interest comprises.

Any proposed operative procedure (such as placing a feeding tube) should trigger the same process.

Speech and language therapists may help with decision making for patients with dysphasia by assessing level of comprehension, or explaining common procedures (such as PEG insertion) with picture cards.

Disturbed behaviour

The commonest scenario for apparent 'objection' to treatment is a patient who is confused—by which we mean delirious, demented, or psychotic. This may manifest itself as agitation, aggression, shouting, wandering, and interference with medical devices such as drips, feeding tubes, or urinary catheters. There may be interference with other patients.
- Make a diagnosis—from the mental state examination (alertness, evidence of hallucinations or delusions, speech, cognition) and a third-party premorbid history.

- Identify any underlying medical conditions—infections (temperature, white cell count, C-reactive protein, focal signs such as sputum or abnormal urinalysis), drugs, hypoxia, heart failure.
- Identify any aggravating factors—pain, constipation, urinary retention, illusions, or misinterpretations (cot sides or prison bars?), fear.
- Nurse in a light, quiet environment, away from other patients if possible, avoid confrontation or threats (they never work), maximize sensory awareness if possible (sit out, glasses, hearing aid).
- Avoid sedative drugs if possible. These are effective at relieving anxiety and psychotic symptoms. If these are driving disturbed behaviour then use drugs. If we are dealing with disorientation and bewilderment in someone with dementia, then short of sedating someone to the point of immobility ('chemical strait jacket') they are unlikely to help.
  As a last resort be guided by the drugs in Table 6.1.
- In the UK psychiatrists are reluctant to use the Mental Health Act in these circumstances, but may do so, and they may need to be consulted about diagnosis and management.
- Best interest in these circumstances is represented by those treatments necessary to maintain the safety of the patient, other patients, and staff, and to address the underlying medical condition.

Table 6.1 Drugs for emergency control of severely disturbed behaviour

Patient group	Try first	Try second	Maximum dose in first 6 h
Already on depot/regular high-dose antipsychotics	Lorazepam 2 mg IM	Repeat lorazepam, then try haloperidol 5 mg IM	Lorazepam 4 mg + haloperidol 18 mg
Acute alcoholic withdrawal	Lorazepam 2 mg IM	Repeat	Lorazepam 8 mg
Frail elderly or severe respiratory disease	Haloperidol 2.5 mg IM	Lorazepam 1 mg IM	Lorazepam 4 mg + haloperidol 10 mg
Highly aroused, physically robust, adult	Lorazepam 2 mg IM + haloperidol 5 mg IM	Repeat	Lorazepam 4 mg + haloperidol 18 mg

Cardiopulmonary resuscitation

The usual principles should apply—except that CPR and DNR orders have got caught up in a welter of rather ill-informed press and political opinion.

The main issue is futility. Success rates to discharge after CPR attempts on coronary care units are about 50%. On general medical wards, they are perhaps 5%. Resuscitation is successful when cardiac arrest is due to ventricular tachyarrhythmias or ventricular fibrillation, which most often occurs shortly after MI.

A long list of other conditions is associated with poor (or negligible) chances of success. These include:

- severe stroke
- systemic sepsis
- severe metabolic derangements
- renal failure
- disseminated malignancy
- severe anaemia
- severe lung disease
- pulmonary embolism
- 'severe general frailty'.

In these cases death is not due to an acute arrhythmia, and CPR is futile. For example, in severe stroke death is due to brain damage, or oedema, raised intracranial pressure and tentorial herniation, pulmonary embolism or sepsis.

People with cerebral vascular disease often have coronary artery disease as well. If primary neurological death is not expected, and there are no overwhelming comorbidities or complications, there is no reason to expect that people with mild or moderate stroke might not benefit from CPR if they collapse unexpectedly with cardiac arrest. In these cases we adopt the 'presumption of active treatment' unless we have information to the contrary.

The patient may have told you that they would not have wanted a CPR attempt. They are quite at liberty to do so under the general rules of consent. In some cases you may like to ask. We feel that it is unduly worrying to approach all patients about their wishes routinely, although a general information sheet might be used. The issues are generally not well understood, and patients may feel they are being told they are going to die, or may fear they are not valued, or might be denied other treatments. Some people are more open to these discussions than others, and things are changing rapidly as the issues are aired in the press and on television.

For patients who are not able to give their own opinions, we can ask family or close friends what the patient would have wanted were they able to say. This information can often be appended to discussions about other things. Avoid the trap of asking the family what they want. It is the patient's best interest that concerns you. This is informed by what the family say, but not determined by them. Some people value life almost at all costs (e.g. orthodox Jews and Muslims).

Dementia, in particular, is a distressing condition, and you should think very carefully about resuscitation attempts on anyone with moderate dementia or worse.

UK government and British Medical Association guidance is that all DNR orders should be discussed with patients and/or their relatives. This raises a difficult barrier to the issuing of appropriate DNR orders. A resuscitation attempt that is not in a patient's best interest constitutes an assault, and is probably illegal (although this has never been tested by the courts). The likelihood that discussions would be unduly distressing is perhaps one good reason for forgoing them.

Drips and feeding tubes

The balance sheet of potential goods and potential harm is given in Table 6.2.

In each case, the pros and cons will be differently balanced. Some will vary with individual opinions. This emphasizes the importance of trying to respect autonomy.

The main problem in deciding about the desirability of inserting a gastrostomy tube is *uncertainty*, about:

- *Outcomes*. Patients admitted with swallowing problems, which do not recover within a couple of weeks usually have had severe strokes. We know that for patients with total anterior circulation strokes at least 60% will be dead within a year; 4% will recover to independence (or fewer, if we exclude patients with initially severe deficits, which recover quickly).

- *How people feel about the value or worth of the likely outcomes*. Most people (but not all) consider life with a severe stroke to be at least as bad as death. We are relatively poor at predicting which people will do well (on the basis of clinical features or scores based on multivariate prediction models).

- *The quality of the evidence on which we have to base decisions*. If someone has written an advanced directive (living will) that precisely described the circumstances that pertain, there is little difficulty. Most have not. We are usually dependent on what family or friends say the person would have said were they able to say—based on what they said before, or what they think they would have said before.

Table 6.2 Benefits and burdens balance sheet for feeding decisions

Potential good	Potential harm
Relieve thirst and hunger	Risk of death or complications during insertion of PEG
Prolong life	Prolong the process of dying
Ensure best chance of making a recovery	Survival in a distressing, highly dependent state
Minimize muscle catabolism, preserving muscle mass	
Ease of nursing	

An alternative way of looking at the problem from the standpoint of 'best interest' and autonomy is to consider what the individual would give up to achieve what they want as a final outcome:

- If we want to give people their best chance of a good recovery, we should feed as many people as possible, in order not to miss those who do well despite initially poor signs.
- If the individual had expressed strong feelings about not surviving in a dependent state, they might be willing to trade the small chance of a good recovery for the avoidance of the much larger probability of surviving but being dependent.

If the patient is in a position to give an opinion, it can be discussed with them (albeit a very difficult discussion). In the end we are usually left with trying to make the best of incomplete and uncertain information. We could try to quantify the options more using formal decision analysis— but this is pretty rough and ready, and rarely done (see Ebrahim, S. and Harwood, R. H., 1999, *Stroke: epidemiology, evidence and clinical practice*, 2nd edn, Oxford University Press, p. 103).

Strictly, the arguments for and against gastrostomy feeding hold for nasogastric feeding, and IV or SC fluids (except that these options have forced time-limited reviews, as cannulae must be re-sited and tubes replaced from time to time).

Experience shows that most patients, in whom feeding tubes are inserted after difficulties deciding, die within a few weeks. This suggests we tend to err on the side of intervention.

Tube feeding is legally a 'medical treatment'. Ordinary feeding by mouth is not. If we are not feeding someone, or intending to do so, it is probably illegal to deny them free access to food and drink, even if their swallow is 'unsafe'. Clearly if any attempt at swallowing leads to distressing aspiration, it cannot be considered in anyone's interest. Most likely the patient would not want to try after one bad experience. However, if able to say, that should be up to the patient. Sips of water are unlikely to cause undue problems. In any case, mouth care is especially important for any patient who is not swallowing.

BMA guidelines suggest that decisions to withhold or withdraw feeding or hydration should be subject to a second consultant opinion. This would be desirable in an ideal world.

Antibiotics for intercurrent infections

If someone is inevitably about to die, antibiotics serve no purpose, unless they are intended to relieve distressing symptoms. They will not usually form part of good terminal care.

The same principles of benefit, burden, and autonomy should underlie decisions to commence antibiotic treatment (implicitly at least—the framework should be held in mind even if the process is not explicitly followed).

Antibiotic treatment for pneumonia is perhaps best thought of in probablistic terms rather than the more usual black and white. It is not a matter of 'active treatment—survival' vs. 'no active treatment—death'. Rather, '20% chance of survival without treatment' vs. '60% chance of survival with treatment'.

This is important because one unfortunate consequence of opting not to treat intercurrent infections on the grounds that the patient is terminally ill, is that the patient survives, but is further (unnecessarily) debilitated.

It should also be remembered that antibiotics have a downside as well, especially in wards where *Clostridium difficile* is endemic. Colitis associated with this produces a debilitating, long-lasting and difficult-to-treat diarrhoea that severely undermines quality of life and rehabilitation prospects.

Who should to talk to whom

If a patient is able to do so, information and explanations should be directed at him or her. Decisions should be made by the person to whom they apply. Who else they want told, or to help or support them in making decisions (even a spouse or children), is up to them. You should not get yourself in the position of telling relatives something that you have not told a patient who is in a position to be told.

An extreme view of confidentiality does not represent good practice either, however. Strictly, we should say nothing to anyone about a patient's health state except to the person themselves, without their permission to do so. Confidentiality has to be traded-off against pragmatism and courtesy.

If a patient is severely ill, unable to communicate or otherwise speak for themselves, naturally close relatives will be concerned and want to know what is going on. Family members may be the only source of important information about someone's medical past, and their likely wishes.

If no family is available, do not forget other sources of useful information: GPs, district nurses, neighbours, wardens (of warden-aided flats), and social services. Watch out for visitors.

Taking the lead on decision-making has traditionally fallen to doctors, but there is no particular reason why this should be so. Sometimes a problem can be introduced by one professional and followed up by another, if a difficult decision needs to be broken gently, if time is needed to think the problem through, or consult others. Senior medical staff should be available and willing to support others in this role.

Summary

1. Consent must be gained for any examination, investigation, or treatment. It may be implicit or explicit, written or verbal. For consent to be valid, sufficient information must be given for a decision to be made.
2. Assume that someone is capable of giving consent unless you can show otherwise.
3. Capacity to consent requires that the person understands the proposed treatment, can retain and weigh up the information to come to a decision, and can communicate it.
4. If someone does not have capacity, act in their best interest. But first make sure you know what that best interest is, by asking people who might be able to give the information you need.
5. If a decision is to be made, first consider feasibility—Do the potential benefits outweigh the potential burdens? Then consider desirability—What does the patient want you to do, or what would the patient have wanted you to do?
6. Following a stroke, patients may not have capacity to consent, or be able to tell you what they want because of drowsiness or coma, confusion, or communication problems.
7. Many severely affected patients will die. Best interest is not necessarily served by aggressive intervention. But it might be. The trick is to determine which, and this can be hard.

Chapter 7

Terminal care

Diagnosing dying

Can we predict death?

Knowing that someone is going to die is useful, even if nothing can be done to avert it:

- Families forewarned can gather and are prepared for the worst.
- Healthcare staff can avoid futile and meddlesome treatments.
- We can concentrate on symptom relief.
- It may be possible to arrange a discharge home for terminal care if that is what everyone wants.
- Families may be more upset about a death that was not expected and about which they had no warning, than being told that death is likely in someone who subsequently recovers. There is a subtle balance between not extinguishing hope and not raising expectations. A useful aphorism is to 'hope for the best, but prepare for the worst'.

We are fairly good at recognizing that someone is about to die when they have disseminated cancer, multiple organ failure, or the later stages of neurodegenerative diseases. For other conditions it is more difficult, including stroke, heart, and respiratory failure.

All other things being equal, prolonging life is a good thing. However, we can sometimes misjudge what is for the best:

- We may be overoptimistic and intervene too vigorously when death is probable.
- We can fall foul of a self-fulfilling prophesy—not treating someone because we think they are dying, and they die for lack of a treatment that would otherwise have saved them.
- Sometimes palliative and potentially curative approaches must proceed together. We may still want to attempt life-prolonging treatment when the chances of success are small, but not completely hopeless. However, we may have to treat many people unsuccessfully to save one life, which may not be justified if the treatment is unpleasant, uncomfortable, or compromises dignity.

Can we predict death after stroke?

No single feature, or prognostic score, determined soon after stroke onset, is sufficiently accurate to allow us to predict death (or survival) with certainty in an individual patient.

A number of clinical features are associated with a poor outcome (Table 7.1). However, there is a difference between saying that a feature, such as unconsciousness, is a poor prognostic sign, and saying that everyone with that feature does badly. For example, the 1-month mortality from primary intracerebral haemorrhage is 50%, worse than the average for stroke. But we can't conclude that everyone with a bleed dies.

The best way of describing the ability of a piece of information (feature, test result or score) to predict an outcome is to calculate:

- The sensitivity (in this case, the proportion of people who die who have the bad feature).
- The specificity (the proportion of people who survive who do not have the bad feature).

There is always a trade-off between the two.

Scores must have a high specificity if we assume that it is worse to predict someone is dying, who goes on to survive (because we may falsely opt to withdraw treatments). To achieve satisfactory specificity (say 95%), in practice sensitivity is no better than 33%. That is, we fail to identify most of the people who will die. If we want to identify all those who will die, we will be too gloomy for many who will survive.

In general we are better at spotting people who will do well, than who will do badly. Some apparently poor prospects surprise us by recovering.

That said, we must make realistic and humane management plans for dying patients. A deeply unconscious patient a few days after a stroke is not likely to survive. IV hydration may be necessary to temporize, while nature takes its course towards death or improvement. 'Primarily palliative' care may be appropriate. However, the uncertainty should be acknowledged, and the decision may be reversed if they improve unexpectedly. This may look like indecision and prevarication, but it is inevitable (and right).

Sometimes doctors and other health professionals will 'get it wrong'— patients will be put through procedures (e.g. feeding tube insertion) or other life prolonging interventions only to die a few days later, or will survive and remain dependent and miserable. This is not necessarily bad care, but due to the unpredictable nature of the disease.

Some other patients 'fail to thrive' or 'turn their head to the wall' after initial survival. Beware the possibility of severe depression, undiagnosed physical comorbidity, or complications, but consider if these patients too are dying, and offer sympathetic symptom control.

Table 7.1 List of features after stroke associated with increased risk of death

Unconsciousness
Intra-cerebral haemorrhage
Total anterior circulation stroke (large middle cerebral artery infarct)
Dysphagia
Gaze palsy
Breathing abnormalities
Heart disease
Severe comorbidity or pre-existing disability
Hyperglycaemia
Pyrexia
Atrial fibrillation
Delirium

Palliative care in stroke— is there a problem?

Many stroke patients die fairly quickly from their strokes, and this will affect the type and nature of palliative care that is appropriate.

The UK Regional Study of Care of the Dying described the experience of symptoms in people dying from stroke (see Box 7.1). Nearly half of people certified as dying 'of a stroke', however, did so a month or more after it occurred. Many symptoms were reported (Table 7.2). Pain, confusion, low mood, and incontinence were particularly common—although we cannot tell which problems were due to the stroke and which were due to comorbidity.

Palliative care is no more of an issue in stroke than other life-threatening conditions, except that stroke has less well-developed support systems than others, cancer in particular. There is less provision for counselling time, and a less developed interface with home care.

Alleviating distressing symptoms is a good thing in its own right. If death is not thought to be imminent, there is a tension between achieving this (with drugs, at least), and an holistic strategy for longer-term health.

Doctors who work with older people are suspicious of symptomatic drug treatments for good reason. All drug treatments carry a burden of side-effects, inconvenience, interaction, and compliance problems. Symptoms may be self-limiting, but the drug treatment continued long after it is needed. Geriatricians usually stop as many drugs as they start.

Box 7.1 The Regional Study of Care of the Dying

- Families and carers of 3696 people who died in England in 1990 were surveyed, about 10 months after the death. They were asked to recall problems during the last year of the person's life. Stroke was the main cause of death for 237.
- Respondents were spouses (20%), siblings or children (37%), other relatives (11%), friends (11%), and professionals (20%). Nine per cent of patients were under 65, and 38% over 85; 12% died within 24 h of the stroke, 18% between a day and a week, and 22% between a week and a month; 11% died at home; 19% spent all of their last year in a hospital, residential or nursing home.
- Respondents reported that hospital doctors and general practitioners tried hard to control symptoms, but between a quarter and a half were inadequately relieved; 80% felt that care by hospital doctors or nurses was adequate.

Stroke 1995; **26**: 2242–8.

Table 7.2 Symptoms perceived as problems by carers of people who died from stroke, excluding sudden deaths

	In last month of life (%)	In last year of life (%)
Urinary incontinence	51	56
Pain	42	65
Confusion	41	51
Low mood	33	57
Faecal incontinence	31	38
Poor appetite	29	37
Difficulty breathing	28	37
Constipation	23	46
Poor sleep	22	42
Swallowing problems	20	23
Dry mouth or thirst	20	31
Anxiety	18	26
Pressure sores	17	21
Unpleasant smell	13	16
Nausea or vomiting	12	22
Persistent cough	8	15

Stroke 1995; **26**: 2242–8.

Palliative and terminal care

'Palliating' is 'alleviation without curing'. Strictly, this is what happens in most of medicine. It is not non-treatment, or withdrawal of active treatments. Instead, it is a prioritization of treatments with the aim of relieving distress, minimizing burden related to treatment, and restoring what independence, autonomy, and control is possible in the circumstances.

'Terminal care' is the management of patients in whom the advent of death is felt to be certain, and not far off, and for whom medical effort is wholly directed at the relief of symptoms, and psychological support of patient and family rather than cure or prolongation of life.

The key principles of palliative medicine are:
- Meticulous management of symptoms.
- Open communication.
- Psychological, emotional, and spiritual support of the patient and of those close to them.

The time frame over which palliative care issues occur stretches from a few hours to several months. Four patterns are seen in stroke care that result in death:
1. Severe stroke, leading to rapid neurological death.
2. Complications of stroke, e.g. pneumonia, in the early or recovery phase.
3. 'Stroke presentation' of tumour, inoperable abscess, or subdural haematoma.
4. 'Incidental' stroke occurring in someone dying from another condition, such as cancer or severe heart or respiratory failure.

Symptom control

- Write a problem list:
  - identify each symptom, disability, or problem;
  - understand its importance (how much does it bother you?) and consequences (what does it stop you doing?);
  - note previous successful and unsuccessful treatments.
- Explain each problem:
  - understand how each symptom has arisen;
  - if you can't find a cause, guess the most likely one—is it caused by the primary disease process, comorbid disease, iatrogenic, or other treatment-related problems?
  - are psychological factors or comorbidity exacerbating the problem?
- Treat the treatable:
  - if symptoms can be relieved by curing a pathology, such as a chest infection, give the specific treatment;
  - think broadly and laterally, e.g. agitation may be caused by pain, urinary retention, hypoxia, drugs, or constipation;
  - if the underlying pathology cannot be cured, use a treatment that can be expected to address the mechanism of the symptoms.
- Assess the effect of the treatment:
  - best-guess treatment will not work every time;
  - symptoms may change;
  - multiple causes for the one symptom can cause apparent treatment failure;
  - relief of one symptom may reveal another;
  - progressive diseases will cause new or worsening symptoms over time;
  - stop drugs if you are not sure they are needed—they can always be restarted.
- Anticipate problems:
  - opiates always cause constipation, and often cause nausea;
  - drug withdrawal (opiates, nicotine, alcohol), and commencement (opiates or steroids) can cause agitation;
  - pressure sores are avoidable.
- Decisions about symptom control fall within the general framework of benefits and burdens, patient choice or best interests, and non-discrimination.
- Table 7.3 (overleaf) gives a list of common symptoms, and some approaches to addressing them. There is a specialist Palliative Care Formulary that lists some specialized or unlicensed uses of drugs (see http://www.palliativedrugs.com, which has a searchable symptom list).

Table 7.3 Common (non-pain) symptoms in terminal care

Symptom	Possible causes	Symptomatic treatment
Nausea	Drugs (especially opiates), constipation, raised intracranial pressure, medullary stroke, vestibular disease, hypercalcaemia, hyponatraemia, uraemia, gastric or bowel stasis or obstruction, disseminated malignancy.	Consult a specialist text for logical drug choices. Metoclopramide, cyclizine, haloperidol, levomepromazine, hyoscine, ondansetron, or combinations. Sometimes dexamethasone or benzodiazepines.
Agitation	Pain, constipation, retention, hypoxia, hypoglycaemia, other metabolic disturbance, anxiety, dementia, delirium (and its causes, including drugs)	Specific cause. Trazodone 50–150 mg at night, sulpiride 100–200 mg bd, haloperidol 0.5 mg bd to 10 mg tds, lorazepam 1–2 mg bd
Anorexia	Infection, depression, nausea, pain, constipation, denture problems, sore mouth	Dietary measures (small portions, soft consistency, preferences, supplements, alcohol). Can try prednisolone 10–30 mg od, megestrol 80–160 mg bd
Fitting	Stroke, tumour, infection, uraemia, hyponatraemia, hypoglycaemia	Oral (or nasogastric) valproate, IV phenytoin, rectal carbamazepine, SC midazolam infusion (20–40 mg/24 h)
Insomnia	Pain, noise, depression, nocturia	Specific cause. Temazepam, chlormethiazole, trazodone, or amitriptyline. Ear plugs

Drooling	Dysphagia, facial weakness	Ipatropium bromide (atrovent) inhaler; transdermal hyoscine hydrobromide or glycopyrronium 200–400 µg tds po
Constipation	Immobility, dehydration, drugs, anorexia, hypercalcaemia	Senna 15–30 mg, docusate 200 mg bd, picosulfate 5–10 mg, or movicol 1–8 sachets/day, co-danthramer 2 capsules once at night (increasing up to tds). Consider glycerin suppositories, or enemas.
Sore mouth	Dehydration, mouth breathing, candidiasis, aphthous ulcers, denture problems, gingivitis	Chlorhexidine mouth wash, pineapple chunks, nystatin, or fluconazole for candida, buccal analgesics (benzydamine, bonjela), triamcinclone in orabase for ulcers
Faecal incontinence	Impaction with overflow, disinhibited colon, diarrhoeal disease, laxatives and other drugs, immobility and communication problems	Clear bowels (abdominal X-ray to assess). Pads, prompted toileting, faecal collecting bags. Loperamide/enemas bowel regimen if planning discharge.
Urinary incontinence	Unstable bladder, incomplete emptying/retention, inability to communicate or move	Prompted voiding, pads, sheath, intermittent or indwelling catheter
Breathlessness	Heart failure, chronic lung disease, lung or pleural malignancy, pleural effusion, pulmonary embolism, pneumonia, chest deformity, acidosis, anxiety	Specific cause. Explanation. Fan, nebulized bronchodilator, Opiates ± lorazepam, or hyoscine butylbromide (for retained secretions).

Pain management

- Assess each pain. There may be more than one.
- Unrelieved pain is intensified by insomnia, depression, anxiety, social isolation, and hopelessness. Consider antidepressants as adjuvants to analgesics.
- Get control of the pain quickly. Which drug you choose depends on initial severity. Use oral morphine or SC diamorphine if necessary, and then decide on a regular regimen.
- Give analgesics regularly for constant or recurring pain. Prescribe short-acting, as-required, medication for acute exacerbations ('breakthrough pain') in spite of regular analgesia.
- Always give paracetamol 1 g qds. This may be sufficient to control the pain, if not it will reduce the requirement for stronger and more toxic drugs.
- Next add a non-steroidal anti-inflammatory drug (ibuprofen 400 mg tds, diclofenac 50 mg tds), or a 'weak opiate'. Coproxamol is no stronger than paracetamol. Dihydrocodeine is poorly tolerated by elderly people (delirium, drowsiness, nausea, constipation, malaise). Tramadol (50–100 mg qds) is often better, but can also cause delirium and constipation.
- If this is insufficient, use morphine or diamorphine.
- All patients on strong opiates become constipated—prescribe senna 2 tablets (15 mg) od or bd plus sodium docusate 200 mg bd, or co-danthramer, initially 2 capsules at night. Laxatives may need to be given several times a day.
- 30–50% of patients on strong opiates get nausea—but it is transient (give cyclizine 50 mg tds or metoclopramide 10 mg tds for first week). Drowsiness is also usually transient (few days). Dry mouth is common. Other opiate-induced problems include hallucinations (try a different opiate, or use halperidol), vivid dreams, myoclonus (use clonazepam), gastric stasis, and itch.
- Tolerance is a minor problem. Addiction is defined as an overpowering drive to take a drug for its psychological effects, associated with behaviours such as drug seeking, escalating doses, loss of social control, and neglect of personal hygiene. Addiction does not occur with drugs taken for pain control, and patients can be reassured of this.
- Alternative opiates are fentanyl patches (applied for 3 days at a time, steady state in 12–24 h, less constipating than morphine, but the smallest patch starts at a high dose for frail elderly people); oxycodone (less drowsiness and delirium, fewer dreams and hallucinations, available rectally), and hydromorphone (less drowsiness).
- For neuropathic pain (burning or shooting quality, allodynia—unpleasant sensation of normal stimuli, usually with altered tactile sensation), try amitriptyline (10–100 mg at night), or gabapentin (100 mg tds working up to 1.8 g/day). Other drugs may work, but are difficult to use—seek specialist help. Nerve blocks, transcutaneous electrical nerve stimulation (TENS) or acupuncture are alternatives.
- For central poststroke pain, try amitriptyline or valproate, but it is always difficult to treat.

- Pains that respond poorly or only partly to opiates include:
  - neuropathic pain;
  - bone pain (add a non-steroidal anti-inflammatory drug, radiotherapy);
  - raised intracranial pressure (use dexamethasone, radiotherapy);
  - tension headache (paracetamol, non-steroidal anti-inflammatory drugs);
  - muscle cramp.

Routes of drug administration

- The oral route is often not available because dying stroke patients are either drowsy or unable to swallow.
- Rectal absorption is good. Paracetamol, diclofenac, domperidone, and carbamazepine are available.
- Transdermal fentanyl and hyoscine hydrobromide (1 mg/72 h) are available.
- Transmucosal lorazepam, prochlorperazine, and phenazocin are available.
- SC (use a 22G butterfly needle). Metoclopramide, cyclizine, hyoscine butylbromide, haloperidol, and diamorphine can all be used.
- Syringe drivers are useful, especially in the agonal (immediately pre-death) phase.

Does symptom control hasten death?

- Palliative care intends neither to hasten nor postpone death.
- Good symptom control may extend rather than shorten life.
- If symptom control measures do shorten life, this is permissible in English law if the intention is relief of suffering, rather than expediting death (the principle of double effect, R v Bodkin Adams 1957. An act that is foreseen to have both good and bad effects is legitimate, provided the act itself is good or at least neutral, the good effect is not caused by the bad effect, and the bad is proportionate to the good).
- Motivation and proportionality are hard to judge. If the sole reason for doing something is to hasten death it is both illegal and wrong.

The last few days of life

- Encourage participation by patient's family and friends, in decision making and practical care, according to views and wishes.
- Reassess needs. Look for non-verbal clues of distress (agitation, grimacing, groaning), examine possible sites of pain (mouth, ears, heels).
- Treat distressing symptoms, and stop all other medication. Pain can always be controlled, but sometimes at the cost of drowsiness or continual sleep.
  - use diamorphine SC, intermittently or by syringe driver. If the patient has not had opiates before start at 5–10 mg/24 h. If opiates have been used before, the dose will depend on previous doses, response, body build, and renal function
  - other drugs can be added to a syringe driver according to the clinical situation, and may include:
    - haloperidol (initially 2.5 mg/24 h) for nausea or agitation
    - midazolam (initially 10 mg/24 h) for anxiety or fitting
    - hyoscine butylbromide (60 mg/24 h) for retained respiratory secretions
  - levomepromazine (start at 5–25 mg/24 h), is a powerful anti-emetic and sedative, which may also be analgesic, and can be given SC—sedation is usual with doses above 50 mg/day.
- Prescribe as required medication for anticipated symptoms—agitation, anxiety, pain, convulsions, noisy respiratory secretions.
- Stop routine observations and investigations unless there is a specific problem to solve, which enhances comfort.
- Give medication transdermally, SC, or rectally if the patient cannot swallow.
- Dry mouth is caused by mouth breathing, drugs, and/or poor fluid intake. Parenteral fluids are rarely needed. Dehydration is not painful and patients rarely complain of thirst. Continued hydration may increase the distress of dying. Use local measures to relieve dry mouth. These must be done regularly and assiduously. Relatives can usefully help in doing this.
- If someone is dying and unable to swallow safely, they should not be denied access to oral fluids (or food if they ask for it). While it is legal to withdraw IV or tube hydration, it is probably illegal to deny oral fluids to someone who wants them. Clearly if distressing choking occurs, the patient may revise their wishes, but staff should not otherwise worry about the risk of aspiration.
- Continue skin care and containment of incontinence—use a sheath or pads or a catheter if necessary.
- Assess relatives' needs.
- Consider discharge home.

If the patient is unconscious, or nearly so, and shows no signs of distress, some treatments that are neutral in terms of benefit or harm to the patients can be justified if they help relieve distress in relatives. Examples include a 'cosmetic' SC fluid infusion, hyoscine for excessive respiratory secretions, diamorphine or haloperidol for agitation or restlessness. Beware features such as grimacing or agitation that may indicate undertreatment.

Psychological support— patients and families

- Psychological assessment and management after a stroke is all the more difficult because of confusion, drowsiness, and dysphasia, which are common in patients with severe strokes. In many cases there will be no meaningful verbal communication between the patient and staff.

- By definition, an unconscious patient has no distressing symptoms, physical or psychological. But watch for clues that this is not the case if consciousness is depressed but not completely lost.

- A drowsy patient who is not agitated probably has no distress, but it is difficult to be sure. Hearing is said to be the last of the senses to be lost. Assume that drowsy patients can hear, and welcome attention and company. Don't talk as if they are not there. Reassure relatives that their presence is helpful, even when they seem to be getting little response in return. Encourage staff not to neglect patients because routine observations have been stopped.

- Communication is the cornerstone of effective psychological support. This comprises listening and talking. Good communication saves time, is more satisfying, and less stressful. Tailor the giving of information to the wishes and understanding of the recipient, especially that involving bad news.

- Be empathetic. Empathy is putting yourself in someone else's shoes. If we have not been in a similar situation ourselves, we must use our imaginations. But people differ one from another, so not everyone's feelings and emotions will be the same as your own. Recognize both the distress of dying or seeing a close relative die, and of being in a strange and disempowering environment (hospital).

- Most people fear death. But many older people are remarkably philosophical about it, realize that lifespan is not infinite, and will have seen contemporaries die. If the patient is able to engage, you can assume that they will have thought about their own death in general terms. Many dying patients are aware of what is happening (see Table 7.4). Most understand and accept. However, in the Regional Study of Care of the Dying, patients dying with stroke were more likely to have to work this out for themselves than were cancer patients (who were more often told by professionals). This means that either the professionals did not know, or were reluctant to share the information.

- Some patients use the psychological defence of denial. If this is protective allow it to continue. If it is creating problems it may need to be challenged. Patients or relatives may insist on non-disclosure of the truth to the other party. This is usually counter-productive. Ask them why? Explanations include previous bad experience, protecting themselves, or a mutual wish to avoid distress. Ask what they know already? It is often more than you think. Isolation, mistrust, and lack of knowledge increase fear and anxiety. Ultimately, the doctor's first duty is to the patient who has a right to know. Be aware of the specific parietal lobe deficit of anosognosia (denial of having a stroke), which is 'neurological' rather than psychological.

Table 7.4 Awareness that the patient was going to die in the Regional Study of Care of the Dying

		Stroke %	Heart disease %	Cancer %
Patients	Knew	40	49	76
	Did not know	35	39	16
	Not known	25	12	8
Carers	Knew	57	37	77
	Half knew	22	22	13
	Did not know	22	41	11
Worked it out for themselves	Patients	80	81	42
	Carers	36	42	20

Addington-Hall, J. (1996). In: *Managing terminal illness* (eds. G. Ford and I. Lewin), Royal College of Physicians of London.

- Ignorance can cause fear. Try to find out what the patient or relatives fear most:
  - uncontrolled pain is rare;
  - fear of inappropriate discharge from hospital, or moving between different wards, is common in a health service pressed for bed capacity—if death is likely within a week or two, patients and relatives should be reassured that they should not be moved unless they want to (e.g. to go home, or to a more conveniently located nursing home) (terminally ill patients in the British NHS have a right not to be discharged);
  - if death is less imminent, fear of dependency, confusion, or incontinence may be allayed by convincing practical plans;
  - fear of overintervention and artificial prolongation of the end of life should be allayed by reassurance;
  - how the family will cope, and finances, are common fears—most fears are lessened by being shared even if not fully resolved.
- Anxiety and depression are almost inevitable in alert, cognitively unimpaired patients. However, in the context of stroke alone, these patients are unlikely to die. Patients with dysphasia have the added burden of frustration and the inability to express their feelings or sometimes to understand information given to them. Anxiety, anger, and a bereavement-type reaction are common in acute stroke. Both anxiety and depression are common in the months after a stroke—due to 'adjustment reactions' (the psychological response to unpleasant events), or dysthymia (minor depression), or major affective disorder. Drug therapy for minor depression is disappointing, but dothiepin or trazodone may help. Major affective disorder is hard to diagnose in any severe physical illness. Worthlessness, guilt, and anhedonia are more useful pointers, along with the persistence and severity of the symptoms. Standard SSRI or tricyclic antidepressant drug treatment is used.
- Allow expression of emotion, and make room for cultural and religious beliefs or practices, which you may not share or feel comfortable with.

- Create a sense of partnership in decision making and care giving. Aim for continuity of care. Anything that enables participation, independence, and a sense of control is good.
- Saying 'don't worry' is unhelpful. Reassurance without explanation is unconvincing and can increase anxiety. A counselling approach is better but time consuming. Get the patient or relatives to state what the problems are, and with the help of some technical explanation, what the possible solutions are. The trick is to give at least the impression of having time to take on problems, which you can do by listening to problems and being sympathetic to them.
- Care of dying people is emotionally costly for staff. Team support is important. You must have confidence in your colleagues (of any discipline) and them in you, and be ready to ask their advice.
- Don't exclude young children. Everyone will want to protect them from distress, but they are perceptive, and exclusion and isolation in the long run makes things worse.
- Spiritual pain is rather alien to our current way of thinking about life. Death raises questions of life and its meaning, feelings of guilt and failure about the past, things left undone, failed relationships. Life may seem meaningless. Patients and relatives may be thinking in these terms even if you are not. Acknowledge them if the opportunity arises.

Bereavement

'Bereavement' describes both the experience of grieving, and the time period during which it occurs. Grieving is the feeling of sorrow, and other emotional reactions, after a loss. This is usually seen in its most intense form after a death, but may be seen as a response to other losses after a stroke—including loss of health, function, body image, roles, interests, and relationships.

People respond to loss in different ways. Sometimes this is unpredictable and unexpected—to everyone, the person themselves, those around them, and staff, including yourself. Understanding the process can help them and us. But don't expect to understand everything, nor for reactions to be logical or 'reasonable'. Sometimes the process may seem alien or embarrassing (such as prayers or high levels of visibly expressed emotion), and sometimes it will get personal (anger and complaints directed against staff). You just have to accept this as part of the job. Try to be tolerant and sympathetic, even if that is not how you feel.

Reaction to a death depends in part on what has gone before:

- Sudden unexpected death. There is no preparation, or anticipation, and in general the impact on surviving relatives will be more severe and disruptive.
- Death in the week or two after a stroke. Often there is a period of uncertainty before death, about survival and the prospect of severe disability, and the balance between life-sustaining supportive medical care and terminal symptom control. But this time allows families some time to adjust to the prospect of loss ('anticipatory grief').
- Death from a late complication, recurrence, or other vascular disease—the initial shock and threat to life will have been experienced, and to some extent adjusted to.

Other important contributors include:

- The personality and personality traits of the grieving person.
- Their personal coping abilities, and things that compromise them such as physical and mental illness.
- Things that enhance coping, including family and social support (including cultural and religious influences).
- The nature, characteristics, and closeness of the relationship with the deceased person.
- Their previous experiences of grieving.

Bereavement can bring overwhelming physical and emotional distress, and be frightening and bewildering. Psychological reactions can include:

- anger
- guilt
- anxiety
- sadness
- despair
- crying

Physical responses include:
- fatigue
- sleep disturbance
- loss of appetite
- bodily symptoms.

Guilt may include the feeling that 'everything possible was not done'. Anger can easily be directed at medical and nursing staff, especially if relatives were dissatisfied with, or misunderstood, some aspect of care. Hence an important preventative function is served by good, sympathetic, communicative, terminal care.

There are a number of theories about grieving. Kubler-Ross's groundbreaking idea that grieving people work through a number of stages (numbness, denial, searching, anger, resolution), is no longer thought to be adequate. Phases of grief are recognized, but people may move back and forward through them. They include:

- Shock and numbness—difficulty in taking in information about the death (so it may need to be repeated; and the need for the grieving person to rehearse the details is not endlessly going on about the death).
- Yearning and searching—intense separation anxiety, and disregard of the reality of the loss, which leads to the need to search for the missing person, with inevitable disappointment.
- Disorganization and despair—with depression, distractibility and poor concentration, and difficulty planning for the future.
- Reorganization and recovery.

A bereaved person eventually needs to adapt and reintegrate into the world. This involves:
- Accepting the reality of the loss.
- Experiencing, expressing, and resolving the physical and emotional distress of loss.
- Adjustment to the environment from which the person is missing.
- Redirecting the emotional energy previously invested in the person who died.
- Forming new relationships.

Over a few months the symptoms fade. Health professionals needs to recognize delayed, inhibited, or chronic grief. Of course, by this time events are probably far removed from the hospital stroke ward, but you may come across bereaved people in other contexts, and sometime repercussions come late (requests to discuss what happened, complaints).

A third of bereaved spouses develop significant physical or mental health problems, and are twice as likely as expected to die in the following year. Health consequences are worse if the death is of a young person, if there are low levels of trust, a previous history of psychiatric disease, a perceived lack of support or understanding, or if the relationship with the deceased was overdependant.

Information can be especially short when the death is unexpected. Bereavement support services are usually available locally.

Summary

1. Many stroke patients die, often days to weeks after hospital admission. For some a palliative care approach is appropriate, either alone, or in tandem with supportive management.

2. Although several prognostic markers have been identified after stroke, and several prognostic scores have been developed, none is accurate enough to be very useful in clinical stroke management. However, patients who are deeply unconscious several days after a stroke are unlikely to survive.

3. Carers of patients dying of a stroke report many distressing symptoms, resulting either from the stroke itself, or from comorbid disease.

4. Palliation is the alleviating of symptoms without cure. Palliative care is the prioritization of treatments with the aim of relieving distress, minimizing burden related to treatment, and restoring what independence, autonomy, and control is possible in the circumstances.

5. Multiple and complex symptoms and problems must be meticulously assessed, explained, and whatever curative or palliative treatment is possible used to relieve them.

6. A considerable body of expertise exists in the control of pain and other distressing symptoms.

7. Open explanation and communication is vital, but is often difficult in dying stroke patients, who may be drowsy, dysphasic, or confused.

8. Allowing family to be involved in decision making and delivering practical care is both useful for the patient (and staff) and therapeutic for themselves.

9. Anticipate, identify, and address fears.

10. Grieving is an intense emotional and physical experience. It is often unpredictable, and needs to be managed with tolerance and sympathy, even when reactions appear unreasonable.

Chapter 8

Rehabilitation

What is rehabilitation?

'A restoration to rights or former abilities'.

There are three elements:

- *Re-ablement*—restoration of function, taking advantage of spontaneous recovery, avoiding complications, learning new skills, and making use of aids and appliances.
- *Re-settlement*—the adaptation of the environment to suit the abilities of the person concerned, and maximize their participation.
- *Re-adjustment*—psychological adaptation, changes in goals and ambitions, re-establishing esteem and fulfilment.

And two broad aims:

- To maximize functional ability.
- To increase the number of options that patients and their families have over eventual discharge—which often means making possible a home discharge where the alternative would have been institutional care.

How to approach rehabilitation

- Make a problem list. Identify, break down, and understand problems. This requires a thorough review of the case notes, discussion with the patient about what is happening, what they understand and what they want, and consultation with family or other carers.
- Set goals—these can be:
  - 'high-level goals', where you eventually want to get (e.g. independence walking, discharge home);
  - 'intermediate goals', things that need to be achieved on the way to the higher-level goals (such as standing, or weight transference between legs).
- Intervene therapeutically.
- Review progress, revise the problem list, and repeat the cycle until all goals are met, or a plateau is reached, when we assume that maximum ability has been achieved.
- Make plans to deal with, or compensate for, any remaining problems.
- Continually reconsider the most appropriate location for rehabilitation, and commence discharge planning.

Convene an early meeting with family, including the patient if he or she is able. Discuss:
- What they have already been told, and what they already know.
- Previous abilities, problems, and support.
- The diagnosis and its effects, especially on current abilities.
- Their expectations.
- The likely prognosis.
- Future options:
  - keep all options open for as long as possible—don't make any assumptions (e.g. that institutional discharge will be inevitable);
  - the likely duration of recovery and rehabilitation;
  - broach the possibility of institutional discharge if it looks likely. Suggest that family members visit a few care homes (the local telephone directory is a good place to start). This enables future discussions to be better informed, and starts the process of finding a suitable home.

If the patient was previously living in a care home, useful information about previous abilities and goals (e.g. what abilities are required to enable a return to the previous home) can be gained by telephoning the home.

Problems (Table 8.1)

'Problems' (in the problem list) can be:
- A risk factor or predisposition (e.g. falling).
- A diagnosis or pathology.
- An abnormality of body structure or function (impairment).
- An inability to perform tasks or activities (previously called 'disabilities').
- Restricted participation—problems at the level of the person in a physical and social environment.

The relationship between these, and the place of different interventions and barriers can be seen from Figure 8.1. If any element is missing, opportunities to improve functioning may be missed.

A comprehensive assessment is essential to avoid difficulties and delays later on. Some commonly-occurring issues need specific plans, some of which may be ongoing from earlier in the admission (Box 8.1).

Table 8.1 Impairment, activity limitations, and participation restrictions

Impairments	Activity limitations/disabilities	Participation restrictions
Poor sitting balance	Sitting	Inability to get where needed or desired
Limb weakness	Transferring	Loss of independence—need for help with daily activities
Spasticity/contractures	Walking	Inability to undertake occupation and
Hemianopia	Stair climbing	responsibilities—employment, leisure, domestic
Dysphasia	Continence	Poor awareness of surroundings
Visuospatial problems/neglect	Toilet use	Inability to sustain social relationships
Poor visual acuity	Dressing	Participation in civil responsibilities
Depression/anxiety	Feeding	
Lack of confidence or motivation	Kitchen skills	
Poor memory, concentration,	Washing, bathing, showering	
judgement, problem solving	Behavioural disturbance	
Detrusor instability	Communication problems	
Polyuria		
Breathlessness		
Pain (joints, central)		
Deafness		

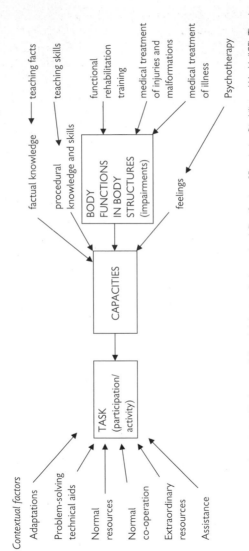

Fig. 8.1 Schematic representation of the WHOs framework for rehabilitation–the *International Classification of Functioning, Disability and Health* (ICF). The aim is to maximise activity and participation. Arrows represent necessary conditions. Devised by Dr Tormod Jaksholt.

Box 8.1 Multidisciplinary rehabilitation headings

- Swallow and nutrition
- Pressure areas/wound care
- Anti-embolic prophylaxis
- Positioning
- Upper limb function
- Movement and mobility
- Standing/transfers/walking
- Safety/falls
- Urinary continence
- Bowels and faecal continence
- Mood and psychological care
- Sleep
- Cognition and perception
- Communication
- Washing and dressing
- Bathing
- Kitchen skills
- Home situation and capabilities prior to admission
- Medication management
- Secondary prevention and life-style modification
- Discharge planning
- Information requirements

Rehabilitation nursing

Rehabilitation nursing may be the single most important element of a rehabilitation unit, requiring flexibility and fine judgement. It involves:

- Using opportunities during daily care to undertake functional activities (getting up, toileting, dressing, walking to the day room or to meals).
- The progressive withdrawal of support as independence and confidence are regained.

This is achieved through:

- Practice of skills or approaches learnt with specialist rehabilitation therapists, and avoidance of poor positioning or inappropriate activities ('the 24-h approach').
- The building of stamina, fitness, and confidence through physical activity.
- Avoidance of complications (pressure sores, joint contractures, venous thrombosis, aspiration, falls).
- Making specialist assessments and management plans for continence and wound care.
- Providing detailed feedback on day-to-day performance.
- Helping to formulate, and working towards, defined goals.
- Providing sufficient help to ensure 'personal maintenance' (hygiene, nutrition, freedom from falls and other danger).
- Being aware of general health, and the ability to react appropriately in a medical crisis.
- Helping to promote psychological adjustment (listening, advising, promoting a positive outlook).
- Being aware of, and managing, patients' and relatives' expectations, in particular where this is manifest as dysfunctional illness behaviour (such as overdependency or overprotectiveness), or overoptimistic goals. Some patients expect to be 'cared for' when they should be learning independence.

Teamwork

- A team is a group of people working together with a common purpose.
- Teams achieve more than individuals working in isolation.
- Each team member should know what they bring to the team, their skills and limitations, and what they are responsible for. Doctors in particular, should not forget that it is their job to get the general medicine right (diagnosis, drug therapy, referral to other specialists).
- Team members should know what other members do. There will be some overlap, but unnecessary replication should be avoided (Table 8.2).
- The team should follow the same approach and strategy 24 h a day, regardless of which discipline they are from.
- Communication is essential, usually via weekly team meetings, when patients are systematically reviewed for problems, abilities, progress towards goals, and when new goals are set and discharge planning undertaken.
- Each involved team member needs to contribute to meetings—and be helped to do so if reticent.
- An objective record of disabilities should be kept, by using standardized scales, or free text.
- Records should be shared or easily accessible to all team members.
- Leadership of healthcare teams tends to be quite informal—meetings need chairing or directing, but decisions are a matter of consensus, and delegation requires persuasion rather than giving orders (see Box 8.2).

Box 8.2 Leadership and team working

Leaders
- Leaders do not just give orders, but enable people to do their jobs better
- Team members enable their leaders to lead, because it is in their interests, makes it easier for them to do their own jobs, and helps to achieve a worthwhile common goal.

Leadership functions
- Integrating information
- Maintaining momentum
- Helping set goals
- Making or confirming decisions
- Developing a vision, identifying new opportunities.

Team working needs
- Clear and agreed roles and duties
- Equal commitment
- Shared responsibility
- Identification and use of individuals' strengths
- Clear communication and sharing of information
- Honest, constructive feedback, including thanks and praise
- Mutual support (e.g. when things go wrong)

Table 8.2 Who does what? Roles of different members of the multi-disciplinary stroke team

Who?	What?
Nurses	Observation, hygiene, basic nutrition and dysphagia management, pressure area care, medication supervision, continence management, counselling, patient and carer education, primary information point for family, continuity, practice of ADL skills, 24-h approach, discharge planning.
Physiotherapists	Assessment and training of motor function, management of abnormal muscle tone and shoulder pain, remediation of mobility disabilities (including trunk control, bed mobility, transfers, walking, and stairs). Other specialist functions may include advice on orthoses, clearing secretions from the lungs, and teaching pelvic floor exercises.
OTs	Assessment and training in personal and domestic ADL, assessment of perceptual abnormalities (neglect, visuospatial problems) and cognition, seating and wheelchair assessment, home assessment visits, advising on and provision of aids and adaptations. Limb splinting.
Speech and language therapists	Assessment and management of neurogenic dysphagia. Assessment and treatment of receptive and expressive language function. Communication training. Provision of communication aids. Advising families and other staff on communication. Support for dysphasic patients and their families.
Doctors	Compiling comprehensive medical formulation—diagnosis, including comorbidity, risk factors, complications. Medical therapy and necessary specialist referral. Depending on local arrangements, co-ordination and overview, communication with patients and families.
Dieticians	Assessment of nutritional needs, and recommendations on specialist diets (including cholesterol and weight reduction). Planning of tube feeding regimens.
Clinical (neuro) psychologists	Assessment of cognitive impairments, perceptual disorders, apraxias, executive functions (planning, decision making), mood disorders, anxiety, adjustment reactions, and emotionalism. Explanation to patients, carers and clinical staff. Direct clinical interventions include cognitive retraining, group or individual psychotherapy, relaxation, and cognitive-behavioural therapy. Supportive counselling and groups for carers.
Social workers	Mainly discharge planning: need for home care support services, meals at home, day centres, institutional care, including respite care. Advice and assessment for financial benefits and institutional care funding. Also may help with suspected abuse, debt counselling, guardianship, and Mental Health Act orders.

ADL, activities of daily living.

Monitoring progress

Progress is best monitored by assessing disability (activity limitation). Three key dimensions are:

- Mobility—transfers, walking, stability and falls, getting to the toilet, stairs, wheelchair use. Include distance achieved, and extent of help and aids required (e.g. walks 20 m with a wheeled Zimmer frame plus one person). Formal scores such as the Rivermead mobility assessment (Appendix 11) are often used by physiotherapists.
- Continence—and other practical elimination issues such as constipation, nocturia, and urinary urgency.
- Behaviour—usually in the context of dementia or a difficult pre-morbid personality trait, but also mood, motivation, engagement, and passivity.

Other aspects such as dressing, and kitchen skills, should be added at the appropriate stage of rehabilitation.

In hospital, a standardized ADL scale (e.g. Barthel Index—Appendix 12) can be used. Ensure sufficient annotation to record the presumed mechanism of outstanding problems. Is the transfer difficulty due to weakness, pain, dizziness, or fear? This may prompt a medical review.

Once home, a wider range of activities should be considered.

Prognostication and prediction—
trajectories of recovery

Trying to anticipate future progress and outcome is required for two reasons:
- Goal setting, and giving of prognostic information.
- To chart recovery and detect deviations, which might indicate complications or the need for reassessment.

Anticipated rate of recovery depends on initial severity. The Copenhagen Stroke Study (Box 8.3) provided detailed weekly information on recovery patterns:
- Recovery in neurological impairments preceded recovery in functional abilities by about 2 weeks.
- Overall 80% of surviving patients had reached their best ADL function within 6 weeks of stroke onset, and 95% within 12.5 weeks.
- Recovery in both impairments and disabilities was most rapid in the *least* badly affected patients (SSS 45–58). Maximum recovery occurred by 8.5 weeks.
- Moderately affected patients (SSS 30–44) had maximum recovery by 13 weeks.
- Severely affected patients (SSS 15–29) had maximum recovery by 17 weeks.
- The most severely affected patients (SSS <15) did not reach a plateau until 20 weeks.

Caveats:
- Do not jump to early conclusions. Some patients regain functional capacities after 6 months—especially, but not exclusively, younger patients.
- Inform patients realistically about the chances of recovery, and negotiate therapy goals (trying to moderate them where they are overambitious—plans can always be remade if things are going better than expected).

Recovery of motor function can be charted in terms of more basic functional tasks ('milestones') agreed by physiotherapists to be important, and which can be assessed very reliably. Table 8.3 illustrates recovery in a series of 368 stroke patients referred for physiotherapy, who survived 8 weeks. This gives a good impression of the rate of recovery in hospital-admitted patients with stroke that compromises functional ability.

Box 8.3 Recovery patterns: the Copenhagen Stroke Study

- 1197 hospital admitted acute stroke patients were assessed weekly using the Barthel index and SSS.
- Evaluation continued until death or discharge, and was repeated 6 months poststroke.
- Initial severity, based on SSS score, was 19% very severe, 14% severe, 26% moderate, 41% mild.
- Neurological impairment after 6 months (among survivors):
  - 11% had severe or very severe deficits
  - 11% had moderate deficits
  - 47% had mild deficits
  - 31% had no or only mild deficits.

Archives of Physical Medicine and Rehabilitation
1995; **76**: 27–32, 399–405, 406–412

Table 8.3 Motor recovery in 368 patients who survived to 8 weeks. Patients were referred within 10 days of their strokes, age range 42–89 years. Items were scored by physiotherapists as able/unable

Task	% achieving task					
	Referral	1 week	2 weeks	4 weeks	6 weeks	8 weeks
Gross body movements						
Lying, turn head	91	98	99	99	99	99
Maintain sitting balance 2 min	59	76	86	91	92	92
Lying, roll on to side	58	73	82	86	89	89
Get up from lying	35	53	64	70	73	76
Stand up to free standing	29	43	52	63	66	71
Transfer bed–chair	27	45	55	63	67	71
Two steps forwards	23	39	48	56	61	66
Two steps backwards	18	33	44	52	57	61
Independent walking inside	14	27	38	45	49	53
Arm movements						
Sitting, clasp and unclasp affected hand	33	47	54	57	60	63
Sitting, place unaffected hand to mouth	27	38	44	49	52	54
Lying, hold arm in elevated position	25	39	45	52	56	56

From *Lancet* 1987; **i**: 373–5.

Mobility

Loss of mobility is fundamental to many of the problems faced in rehabilitation. Mobility disability accounts for at least half of the variation in disability in other areas (if you are immobile, maintaining continence, dressing, kitchen skills, and occupation are difficult).

Impairments contributing to mobility problems include:
• Muscle weakness.
• Balance problems, dizziness, or postural instability.
• Neglect.
• Hemianopia and visual acuity problems.
• Joint instability, contractures, and pain.
• Heel sores.
• Breathlessness.
• Anxiety.
• Psychomotor retardation and advanced dementia.

Each impairment needs identifying, explaining, and treating in so far as is possible. Ask the question 'what is preventing mobility?'. Answering requires communication between medical, nursing, and therapy staff.

Most of the recovery of motor function is spontaneous. The task of rehabilitation is to:
• Facilitate or enhance this process as much as possible.
• To take advantage of recovery by translating it into useful functions.
• To avoid setbacks caused by complications.

Neurophysiotherapy aims to maximize motor function, reduce abnormal muscle tone, promote symmetricality, and teach normal movement patterns. Early standing is used to establish trunk control. Transferring techniques, and the safe use of mobility aids are also taught.

'Deconditioning' is the loss of strength, stamina, cardiorespiratory fitness, balance, and confidence that accompanies acute illness and prolonged disability, especially when associated with subnutrition and infection. Fortunately this can be restored with exercise, and repeated practice at every opportunity is important to achieve this (walking to the toilet, to the day room, the therapy gym).

'Compensation'—using the unaffected limb to overcome limitations imposed by paralysis is a difficult topic:
• Some attempts at compensation for hemiparesis are dysfunctional—such as overactivity in the unaffected side ('pushing'), and must be avoided or unlearned. This occurs in about 10% of patients, and delays functional recovery by up to a month.
• Later, compensation is adaptive. Half of patients surviving with initial severe upper limb paralysis get no useful recovery, yet half get independent in upper limb functional tasks by compensatory use of the other limb.

Walking aids and wheelchairs

Walking aids are used to help increase mobility by:
• Improving stability and balance.
• Compensating for muscular weakness.
• Building confidence.

- Prevention of falls.
- Assisting weight bearing following injuries of the lower extremities.

Types of walking aids:
- Walking ('Zimmer') frames, with or without wheels (Figure 8.2).
- Walking sticks (standard, tripod, or quadpod/quadstick; Figure 8.3).
- Crutches.
- Manual, electric, or companion wheelchairs.
- Wheeled shopping trolleys.
- Electric scooters.

Physiotherapists are trained to select an appropriate walking device and to 'progress' as recovery occurs:
- A walking stick has to be of the appropriate height (the handle reaching the wrist of the patient while he/she is standing). A 'high stick' may be used (in the unaffected arm) to promote equal weight distribution, as an aid to recovery.
- Further training is needed if the stick is going to be used to climb stairs.
- Tripods and quadpods increase the 'base of support' to provide better stability but they are heavier than standard sticks, and can encourage abnormal movement patterns.
- Crutches are not usually used in patients with stroke but are useful for patients with lower limb injuries.
- Four-legged walking frames (Zimmer frames) must be picked up and advanced with every step, and hence are little use for patients with a paralysed arm. They can be useful for patients with truncal co-ordination problems (ataxia).

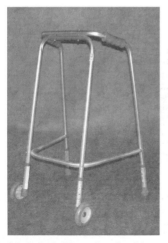

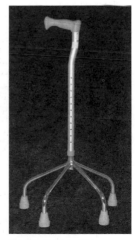

Fig. 8.2 A wheeled Zimmer (or rollator) frame.   **Fig. 8.3** A quad stick.

- Wheeled walkers help the patient to walk faster, but at the expense of stability. The addition of wheels assists in pushing the frame forward without lifting.
- For less disabled patients, three-wheeled delta frames gives good speed and manoeuvrability for those who can control them. The patient can change direction without lifting.

OTs assess the suitability and type of wheelchair and give instruction in their use:

- Wheelchairs may be used indoors though they are often used only for outdoor activity. The companion wheelchair can be folded down to put in a car.
- Motorized wheelchairs and scooters need special assessment.
- Early wheelchair use is controversial. Patients may want the earlier independence (often 'scooting' with the unaffected leg), while therapists worry about the effects on tone and symmetricality.

There is a flourishing private sector for mobility aids and devices. It may not be easy for patients to get good independent professional advice about the suitability of these products. Some local authorities and voluntary organizations run disability assessment centres where patients can try out aids and get advice.

Stairlifts can be very useful, but a safe transfer on and off, good sitting balance, and freedom from blackouts (e.g. fits) are required.

Outdoor mobility

Outdoor mobility requires balance, confidence, and stamina beyond that needed indoors. The terrain is more challenging, and may be unpredictable. The consequence of falling or otherwise running into trouble are all the more serious.

- One problem is fear—so people perform below the level they are capable of. Encouragement and supervised practice can provide some easy gains, and are most easily delivered in home-based rehabilitation schemes.
- Crowded environments are worrying for people struggling with postural stability. Hospital corridors can be used to start with. Supermarkets are another opportunity, choosing an off-peak time initially.
- Another strategy is to upgrade the walking aid—for example, using a stick indoors and a delta frame outdoors.
- Cars (as driver or passenger) and community disabled transport schemes have the potential to increase participation even when residual problems would make independent outdoor mobility impossible. Practice getting in and out of a car may be required.
- A mobile phone can alleviate some of the consequences of a fall or other mishap while out.

Spasticity

Spasticity is excessive, inappropriate, and involuntary muscle activity resulting in stiffness. Secondary biomechanical factors (muscle shortening and joint stiffness) are also important. Established spasticity hinders normal movement, and may cause pain, spasms, hyper-reflexia or clonus and contractures.

Physiotherapy tries to prevent or reduce spasticity, and must commence very early on. Initial changes can occur within a few days of a stroke, and once established are hard to reverse. Achieving some active movement helps prevent spasticity. Splinting of the hand and wrist can help, and may even improve whole arm function, truncal tone, and gait. Patients can be taught methods to lengthen forearm muscles, reducing wrist and finger flexion. Poor positioning, pain, constipation, urinary retention, and pressure sores exacerbate spasticity.

Increased tone in the lower limb hinders stepping through of the unaffected leg (as it won't 'release'). In the upper limb the increased tone pulls the elbow, wrist, and fingers into flexion. Preventing a completely paralysed hand from contracting is difficult. This can affect dressing, and make hand hygiene impossible. Sometimes a spastic leg (holding the limb in extension) allows weight to be born for transferring or walking. However, the extended (plantar flexed) foot tends to drag and cause falls. An ankle–foot orthosis may help.

Anecdotally, the prevalence of badly contracted limbs and 'circumduction gait' has decreased over recent decades with improvement in therapy techniques and delivery.

Drug treatment is generally disappointing. The risk in reducing muscle tone with drugs is that weakness is made worse, and function reduced. Baclofen (start at 5 mg bd or tds, increase up to 20 mg tds), tizanidine, or dantrolene (monitor liver function tests) are sometimes useful. All can cause drowsiness or confusion.

Botulinum toxin injections can be used to reduce abnormal tone without systemic side-effects or inducing weakness.

In severe cases of contracture, often indicating poor previous management, surgical tendon releases can be considered.

Dexterity

Hand function recovers last and least. Intensive arm training has some effect, but the effect is fairly small. Persisting loss of dexterity, especially in the dominant hand, is a particular problem.

The main therapeutic technique is repeated practice of functional tasks and avoiding disuse. This maintains sensory input, flexibility, and muscle strength.

Continence

Continence can make or break the chances of a successful discharge.

Urinary

Half of patients admitted to hospital are initially incontinent of urine.

- About half of these have detrusor hyper-reflexia (an unstable bladder, one which contracts before it is full and when the patient does not want it to, a failure of inhibition of detrusor contractions).
- Frontal lobe lesions sometimes result in an extreme form of this—urinary precipitancy, where there is no warning at all.
- A quarter have retention.
- The other quarter have normal bladder function (on cystometry). Presumably their problems are due to awareness, communication, immobility, and lack of access of suitable aids (urinals, commodes, or toilets).

In each case the abnormality may be due to the stroke or comorbid pathology.

- 20% of stroke patients have continence problems before their stroke.
- 20% of people over 70 have detrusor instability in the absence of stroke—due to idiopathic primary detrusor instability, prostatic enlargement, oestrogen deficiency, stones, or bladder cancer.
- Incomplete bladder emptying is most often due to prostate disease, faecal impaction, or anticholinergic drugs, but a proportion have idiopathic detrusor underactivity, including some women.
- Dementia is associated with lack of awareness, communication difficulties, bladder instability, and sometimes behavioural problems.

Management:

- Perform urinalysis, and if abnormal send urine for culture. If there is haematuria this may require investigation. If there is infection, treat it.
- Measure the postvoid residual volume, preferably by ultrasound scanner, by catheterization if ultrasound is unavailable.
- Ensure a reasonable fluid intake—aim for 2 litres a day plus what comes in food, and avoid caffeine, but caffeine withdrawal symptoms can be unpleasant (concentrated urine and caffeine irritate the bladder).
- If possible complete a 3-day frequency-volume chart. This will give an idea of functional bladder capacity (low, often less than 200 ml, in instability), total urine output, and the day–night split of output. If the patient is incontinent into pads, these can be weighed to estimate voided volume.
- Add an anticholinergic if the residual volume is less than 100 ml. The newer bladder-selective drugs provide the best balance between efficacy and side-effects (mainly dry mouth and heartburn). Tolterodine XL 4 mg od, or propiverine 15 mg bd-qds are best. But none of these drugs is dramatically effective. In trials, cystometric bladder capacity increased from about 200 ml to 250 ml (normal capacity 400–600 ml, a little lower in an older person).
- Try prompted voiding every 2–3 h.
- Vaginal oestrogens sometimes relieve urgency and can be a helpful adjunct (creams are messy—use 'Vagifem'® vaginal tablets).

- Consider the possibility of genuine stress incontinence (leakage on raising abdominal pressure without detrusor contractions). The first line treatment is pelvic floor re-education. Pelvic floor contraction helps inhibit unstable detrusor contractions, so there is some benefit from pelvic floor exercises regardless of diagnosis. There may also be an associated cystocoele, which needs diagnosing and appropriate management.
- If there is retention, try a Queens Square Bladder Stimulator (a vibrating massaging device), intermittent catheterization, or an alpha-blocker (doxazosin 1 mg increasing to 4 mg od, terazosin 1 mg increasing to 5 mg od—both need titrating up to avoid postural hypotension, but can be co-indicated as antihypertensives, or tamsulosin MR 400 μg od, which is uroselective and has less effect on BP).
- If unsuccessful optimize containment:
  - For men try a sheath catheter (penile size should not matter).
  - Otherwise try pads—these have a capacity up to 900 ml, but if saturated are heavy (900 g).
  - Indwelling catheters are a last resort—they always get infected, block, or bypass due to bladder spasm. An anticholinergic may be needed for this. Do not shrink from a 'trial of catheter' if that is what the duly-informed patient wants, and it is the only way to get someone home. The usually well-justified reluctance to use catheters can be taken too far.
  - Consider a suprapubic catheter if intended as long-term— they are more comfortable and less prone to infection.

Other urinary symptoms can be equally troublesome, in particular urgency and nocturia. The need for multiple transfers on to the commode or trips to the toilet at night is a major falls risk and can place considerable strain on a spouse or cohabiting carer:
- Make continence as easy as possible—use regular prompted voiding, or provide urinals.
- Urgency almost always means detrusor instability, but can sometime indicate incomplete bladder emptying. Do a bladder scan and then give an anticholinergic.
- Nocturia can indicate:
  - Unstable bladder—should be detectable from frequent low volume voids on the frequency-volume chart.
  - Nocturnal polyuria—night-time (8 h while asleep) output should be less than one-third of total output. Normal urine output rate is 70–100 ml/h—depending on fluid intake. The normal young adult circadian rhythm in ADH-vasopressin secretion reduces this to 35 ml/h during sleep. Causes of nocturnal polyuria include diabetes, alcohol consumption, oedema, lithium therapy, heart failure, hypercalcaemia, and, most commonly, age-related nocturnal polyuria. If the latter, this is a combined loss of diurnal variation in vasopressin secretion and partial renal unresponsiveness to it (i.e. partial cranial and partial nephrogenic diabetes insipidus). Try giving chlorthalidone 100 mg bd, decreasing to 50 mg od after a month (this has a paradoxical antidiuretic action by sensitizing

renal tubules to ADH). It often cuts night-time output by about
a half. Frusemide 40 mg in the morning sometimes helps, but causes
urinary problems of its own. Desmopressin 200–400 µg given
6 nights in 7 sometimes works, but is often disappointing in practice.
Moreover, in the UK it is not licensed for use in people over 65,
who are more prone to hyponatraemia, and who are often
hypertensive.
- Insomnia—ask about pain, anxiety, depression.
- Incomplete bladder emptying—will need relieving, medically
  (alpha-blockers), surgically (transurethral resection of the prostate)
  or with a catheter (intermittent if possible).

Faecal incontinence
- This is very common in the early period after severe stroke.
- In the longer term, persisting and uncontrolled faecal incontinence
  is a major barrier to discharge home.
- Seek a cause (Box 8.4), but don't expect this to be easy.
- Many patients are constipated. The rectum is a mucus-producing
  organ, and a hard faecal mass stimulates its production, which then
  leaks out as 'spurious diarrhoea'. A rectal examination, and often
  an abdominal X-ray is required. Treatment is with laxatives (senna
  15–30 mg/day, sodium docusate 200 mg bd), or enemas. Avoid
  constipating drugs, and ensure adequate fluid intake. Later on
  encourage mobility and adequate dietary fibre.
- A disinhibited colon may recover with time. Apart from excluding
  constipation, there is nothing to be done in the acute phase. Later
  on try to anticipate bowel opening (keep a bowel chart). If a discharge
  depends on continence, initiate a bowel regimen (loperamide
  2–16 mg/day) to induce constipation, then arrange enemas two
  to three times a week for a controlled bowel evacuation. Patients
  often find this unpleasant. Otherwise, ensure adequate containment
  (pads), and that they are changed quickly if soiled.
- Be aware of drug-induced diarrhoea (laxatives, iron, proton pump
  inhibitors, and metformin).

Box 8.4 Causes of faecal incontinence

- Constipation with overflow incontinence
- Disinhibited 'neurogenic' colon
- Diarrhoea
- Laxatives or other drugs
- Diminished level of consciousness or unawareness
- Immobility
- Severe dementia

Mood

- One to four months after a stroke 10–20% of survivors are depressed and a quarter anxious. Over half will recover within a year.
- Depression is strongly associated with physical disability and somatic illness. It is most likely due to loss of abilities, and threats to life, future independence and ambitions, than anything more 'neurological'.
- Emotional lability, usually inappropriate crying, in the absence of a sufficiently strong stimulus, is not the same as depression, but responds well (and quickly) to both SSRIs and tricyclic antidepressants. It affects about 15%, and is often triggered by emotionally laden questions. The crying is distressing despite its inappropriateness.
- Assessing depression in these circumstances is difficult. Features include:
  - inability to concentrate
  - irritability
  - insomnia
  - hopelessness
  - worry about the future.
- Somatic features, such as fatigue, sleep disturbance, poor appetite, weight loss, and constipation are too non-specific to be useful in isolation. Inability to enjoy things or undertake previous activities is as likely due to the physical effects of stroke as a mood disorder.
- Dysphasia may make assessment almost impossible.
- Depression will often present as a possible explanation for a problem such as lack of motivation, or failure to make progress anticipated.
- Sometimes the diagnosis will be an 'adjustment reaction' (the understandable psychological response to unpleasant circumstances). This fluctuates day to day, and is distractible.
- Major affective disorder is hard to diagnose in any severe physical illness (Box 8.5). Worthlessness, hopelessness, guilt, and anhedonia are useful pointers, along with the persistence and severity of the symptoms. To make a diagnosis of depression symptoms must persist for at least 2 weeks.
- Therapy is largely unevaluated. All the things that comprise good multidisciplinary care should help (a positive and purposeful approach, identifying and tackling practical problems, and time to talk).
- Often we resort to a therapeutic trial of antidepressant drugs. But remember these drugs have side-effects. SSRIs are the current favourites, but their advantages over tricyclics are overstated. They are probably at least as likely to cause falls as tricyclics, and various other problems can be seen, including nausea, anxiety, hyponatraemia, delirium, and extrapyramidal movement disorders. There is little to choose between types. Fluoxetine (20 mg od) is cheapest, followed by paroxetine.
- Lofepramine (start at 70 mg od, increase up to 210 mg/day in split doses), trazodone (50–200 mg at night), and dothiepin (50–150 mg at night) can be also useful, the latter two where anxiety or agitation are problematic, but have anticholinergic side-effects and are more cardiotoxic than SSRIs.
- Make sure drugs are stopped if they are ineffective, but give them a decent trial (3 weeks) after titrating up to full dose.

Box 8.5 Diagnostic criteria for major affective disorder

- Usually:
  - depressed mood—varying little from day to day, or with circumstances, but often worse in the morning;
  - loss of interest and enjoyment, loss of response to enjoyable activities, events, or surroundings;
  - reduced energy, increased fatigability after minimal effort, diminished activity.
- Commonly:
  - reduced concentration and attention;
  - reduced self-esteem and self-confidence;
  - ideas of guilt and worthlessness;
  - bleak and pessimistic view of the future;
  - ideas or acts of suicide or self-harm;
  - disturbed sleep (early morning waking by more than 2 h from usual);
  - diminished appetite, weight loss of >5% in a month;
  - loss of libido.
- Atypical features:
  - anxiety, agitation;
  - hypersolomnence;
  - psychomotor retardation.
- Lasting more than 2 weeks

ICD-10 Classification of Mental and Behavioural Disorders,
WHO, 1992

Communication

Dysphasia (aphasia) and dysarthria affect 20% of stroke survivors each. Half of these will still be dysphasic 6 months after a stroke, although dysarthria tends to recover.

Assess both understanding and expression. Be aware of other problems that might complicate an assessment of language function—deafness, concentration, visual problems, cognitive impairment, depression.

Simple tests:
- Assess spontaneous speech.
- Follow simple motor commands: close eyes, show tongue.
- Questions with yes/no answers.
- More complex, two- and three-stage motor commands.
- Object naming, increasingly difficult (e.g. watch, strap, buckle, winder, hands).
- Repetition.
- Describing a picture.
- Reading and writing.

Discuss functional communication (ability to make needs known, or to follow or co-operate with requests) with other team members.

Speech and language therapists will give a detailed and systematic assessment of the language problem, which can be useful in helping the rest of the team (and relatives) understand the problem. They can also advise on communication aids (e.g. picture boards), pacing of speech, and non-verbal cues. All staff should have a basic understanding of these.

At least as valuable a function as improving language is the provision of explanation or support. Language disorders are generally not well understood, and may be mistaken for dementia. Severe aphasia is immensely frustrating for both patient and carers. Emotional support, practical advice, and contact with other people with similar problems are all required.

How to talk to someone with dysphasia—see Chapter 3 section on 'Dysphasia (or aphasia)'.

Activities of daily living

OTs and nurses are the key, but teamwork remains important. Dressing is hard if the patient cannot stand up, or is dizzy or breathless.

The approach to solving problems is:

- To identify the activity (or level of activity) required or desired, and set goals.
- Recognize the problems in achieving it, and anticipate how these problems (e.g. limb weakness) may change.
- Identify any aids or adaptations necessary to make the task easier or safer.
- Teach new ways of doing the task. This may involve breaking a task down into smaller steps, practising sequencing, and techniques such as verbalizing if dyspraxic.
- Practise it.
- Identify barriers that other disciplines may help overcome (nocturia due to polyuria or unstable bladder, standing difficulties due to heel sores) and liaise with the appropriate person.
- Assess how the function will be undertaken in the home environment, including work with other professionals, family, or other carers (training in transfers, including using a rotunda or hoist, managing stoma or catheter bags, advice on food and fluids consistencies and safe swallowing tips, or delivering PEG feeds).

These may be backed up by home visiting, or in rehabilitation follow-up.

Falls and fractures

- Falls and fractures are a particular concern after strokes.
- Osteoporosis is common among the older (especially female) population, and is worse in hemiparetic limbs.
- Over half this population will have biochemical vitamin D deficiency, or insufficiency (suboptimal vitamin D levels from the point of view of bone health, with secondary hyperparathyroidism, without overt deficiency). Many stroke patients may benefit from vitamin D supplementation, either:
  - as a 6-monthly or annual IM injection of 300 000 units of vitamin D (ergocalciferol), or
  - a combined high-dose calcium (1 g/day) and vitamin D tablet (800 iu/day)—the evidence for benefit is stronger for regimens including the extra calcium, but the cost is yet more tablets, which are large and sometimes difficult to take.
- Patients with a history of low trauma fracture or kyphosis are candidates for a bisphosphonate (alendronate 70 mg weekly). An alternative is raloxifene, which may have additional protective effects against cardiovascular disease and breast cancer.
- Multifactorial falls prevention should be undertaken:
  - diagnose postural dizziness or syncope;
  - check for postural hypotension;
  - medication review avoiding neuroleptics, sedatives, antidepressants, and hypotensive drugs in the presence of postural hypotension;
  - advise getting up from bed or chair slowly;
  - check for cataracts;
  - up to date glasses;
  - optimize gait pattern and transfer technique;
  - muscle strength and balance training;
  - check for foot problems and arrange chiropody;
  - diagnose and treat nocturia;
  - optimize lighting;
  - minimize environmental hazards.
- Remember that the immediate risk from a fall due to postural hypotension (1–2% risk of hip fracture, 5% risk of other fracture, 10% chance serious injury per fall) is greater than the future risk of stroke from hypertension.
- A patient who is falling frequently may like to try mechanical hip protectors (pants with plastic 'shin-pads' sewn in over the greater trochanters). For those who actually wear them regularly (many find them too uncomfortable), these provide a high level of protection against hip fracture. But they are expensive (£30 a pair), and you need 3 pairs (one on, one in the wash, one for tomorrow).

Higher-order skills

- *Driving (http://www.dvla.gov.uk).* Permitted if safe, 1 month after the stroke. The final decision on granting a licence is with the Driver and Vehicle Licensing Agency (DVLA) in the UK, who may take advice from medical staff involved. The driver's insurer must also be informed, or the insurance may become invalid.
  - Severe disability precluding driving should be obvious to all concerned, but identifying cognitive disabilities making driving unsafe may be more difficult, especially where insight is lacking.
  - A hemianopia precludes driving.
  - Epilepsy regulations hold (for car drivers, a fit within the first 24 h of a stroke can be discounted; otherwise no driving for a year after a fit, or while withdrawing antiepileptic drugs, or for 6 months after complete discontinuation of drugs).
  - Following frequent TIAs, there must be 3 months free of attacks.
  - Heavy Goods Vehicle (HGV) and Public Service (PSV) licences can be restored after at least 12 months if a full and complete recovery from stroke or TIA has been made.
  - Specialist neurological OTs may be able to do a paper and pencil screening assessment (the Stroke Drivers Screening Assessment) to identify those likely to have driving problems.
  - A simulator or test track assessment at a specialist mobility centre may be required (for a fee). These centres can also advise on vehicle adaptation and offer retraining, for example, to rebuild confidence.
- *Exercise, physical activity, and sex.*
  - Graded exercise is encouraged where physically possible, without restriction, not least as part of secondary prevention.
  - Another stroke is unlikely during sex. Staff should make it clear that discussion of sex is legitimate, and someone willing to talk about it identified in advance of the question arising. Sexual problems my reflect fear of another stroke, communication problems, relationship problems, depression, the effects of physical disability or incontinence, or impotence. Barriers caused by physical disabilities might be helped by trying new positions. Suggest (or refer on to) relationship counsellors if necessary, including specialists for people with disabilities (in the UK, e.g. Relate and SPOD).
  - Drugs can cause lack of libido and impotence (including antihypertensives and antidepressants). Impotence may also be caused by comorbid diseases, such as diabetes and peripheral vascular disease.
- *Employment, child care, and adult caregiver skills.* Stroke survivors can do what is possible and safe. Professional staff will often be faced with being asked for advice in areas where they feel they have no specific training. Know your limits, but explore the problems, discuss them at multidisciplinary meetings and think broadly and laterally in suggesting solutions. OTs, employers' occupational health advisers, younger disabled (rehabilitation) services, and local authority disability services will have most expertise in employment matters.

- *Body image.* Facial droop, speech problems, abnormal posture, or gait attract stigma. Able-bodied people tend to 'talk over' people with disabilities rather than talking to them, and may avoid them altogether. Professional staff must try not to fall into the same trap. Psychological readjustment requires restoring self-confidence and esteem:
  - Encourage wearing of own clothes, taking pride in appearance, and using make-up if preferred.
  - Talk to patients as sensible adults.
  - Make compliments and positive comments.
  - Encourage family and visitors to do the same, and point it out if they do not.
  - Communal meals can help.
  - Offer tissues for drooling, glasses, hearing aid.
  - Make sure nails are cut, and shaving done properly.
  - Ensure the privacy that is usually expected for washing and going to the toilet. Avoid commodes if possible.
  - Ensure the availability of appropriate feeding aids, change clothes after food spills.
  - Respect cultural needs and differences.

Where to do rehabilitation

In-patient hospital wards

Conventionally, rehabilitation has taken place on specialist hospital wards (stroke units, or mixed rehabilitation wards). There is good evidence that these improve outcomes—about a 20–30% reduction in risk or death, dependency or institutional care compared with 'standard care' on a general medical ward (Box 3.2).

Some models have mixed acute and rehabilitation stroke wards, acknowledging that the transition from 'acute' to 'rehabilitation' is arbitrary. On the other hand, some aspects of acute care (intensive monitoring, dealing with parenteral infusions) can detract from rehabilitation nursing. So other models separate these functions, while recognizing that staff dealing with acute stroke should be trained in rehabilitation, and adequate therapy provision is made on acute wards to cover this function.

In-patient stroke unit rehabilitation is the current 'gold standard of care' against which innovations must be compared.

Home rehabilitation

If a patient is able to transfer alone, or with the help of a willing carer (to allow them to get to the toilet in the night), and has sufficient cognitive insight and judgement to maintain safety if left alone for a few hours, then home rehabilitation is feasible if there is a service locally. This care divides between 'early discharge' schemes designed to expedite hospital discharge, and longer-term community support and rehabilitation services (see Box 9.1).

Home therapy has some clear potential advantages—such as working on activities in the environment in which they will eventually have to be performed, with the people and resources likely to be available to help, as well as avoiding the unpleasantness of hospital wards and ambulance journeys.

Other forms of 'intermediate care'

In the UK these are defined as short-term rehabilitation schemes, lasting a maximum of 6 weeks, designed to prevent hospital admission, expedite hospital discharge or provide postdischarge rehabilitation after an episode of acute illness. Such care may be provided in residential or nursing homes, and may also include the types of home rehabilitation described above. From the point of view of stroke, the short time-frame limits applicability for the most affected patients, and these models are untested according to the best modern standards of evidence.

Summary

1. Rehabilitation is the process of restoring functional ability after an illness, and then helping the patient to come to terms with ongoing disability.
2. Interventions include preventing or treating pathologies (or complications), relieving impairments, and remediating disabilities, taking full account of the social and physical environment.
3. It is necessarily multidisciplinary, and members should work together as a team, communicating regularly and systematically.
4. Problems should be identified and goals set, in order to evaluate progress and identify complications or setbacks.
5. Rehabilitation should occur in the place most appropriate to the particular problems identified, including at home.
6. Mobility, continence, psychological, and behavioural problems are central to successful rehabilitation, and require expert assessment and management.
7. Broader (occupation, leisure) and higher-level skills (driving, employment) also need attention.

Chapter 9

Discharge

When is it time for discharge?

The time for hospital discharge is when what is needed can be provided elsewhere.

If you are going to stay in hospital it has to be for a purpose—mainly because hospitals are no place to live a life, but also because beds represent a scarce resource. Reasons for being in hospital include:

• Nursing care (feeding, washing, hygiene, basic mobility, protecting pressures areas, avoidance of other complications, delivering medication), especially where care is required unpredictably or intensively 24 h a day.
• Access to diagnostic tests, not available outside hospital.
• Access to medical treatments (usually of complications in this case), not available outside hospital.
• Delivery of rehabilitation.
• Waiting—for tests, treatment, or for home or institutional care to be organized or available.
• Convenience of not requiring multiple trips to hospital for tests or therapy or medical consultations.

Much nursing and rehabilitation can be delivered at home. Increasingly, community services are available that can do this (Box 9.1). This is not an excuse for indiscriminate off-loading of patients. The gold standard for acute and rehabilitation care is an in-patient stroke unit. Any community rehabilitation scheme must match (or exceed) what a stroke unit can provide. This means:

• Multidisciplinary staffing, with OT, physiotherapy, nursing, speech and language therapy and access to dietetics, social work, clinical psychology or mental health nursing if needed.
• Ideally, consultant medical support.
• Therapy support workers, either discipline-specific, or more usually generic rehabilitation assistants.
• Adequate numbers of staff to provide as much therapy as the patient can tolerate.
• Multidisciplinary meetings to communicate, co-ordinate, identify problems, set goals, monitor progress and plan eventual discharge.

Box 9.1 South London Early Discharge Scheme for stroke

- 331 patients (about half the stroke admissions during the study) were allocated to home rehabilitation for three months, or to further hospital care. The criterion for inclusion was ability to transfer from bed to chair independently or with the help of a willing carer. Half the hospital care group were treated on a stroke unit.
- Home care was individualized, with up to one visit per day from each of physiotherapy and OT, plus up to 3 h daily of Social Services generic personal care.
- One year later, there were no differences in outcomes (motor weakness, 5-metre timed walk, disability (Barthel Index), cognition, anxiety and depression, carer strain and satisfaction). On average six days hospital stay per patient randomized were saved.

British Medical Journal 1997; **315**: 1039–44

Is discharge safe?

Consider fitness for discharge at the levels of:
- the person
- their abilities
- the environment.

At the person level, this will mean being 'medically stable':
- In a stable cardiac rhythm, with adequate BP, free from severe heart failure or any life-threatening cardiovascular problems (acute coronary syndrome, tamponade).
- Adequate, and stable, respiratory function.
- Free from acute renal failure, or other severe metabolic derangement such as severe dehydration, electrolyte or glucose disturbance.
- Free from severe infection.
- Able to swallow safely, or having a means of non-oral feeding (i.e. a PEG tube).
- Free from severe debilitating symptoms such as frequent fits, pain, nausea, or breathlessness.

At the level of activities, at a minimum, it will require:
- Ability to transfer from bed to chair, wheelchair, or commode, alone or with a willing and able carer (with a hoist if necessary).
- Continence, or adequate containment.
- Measures to relieve skin pressure.
- Ability, judgement, and insight to avoid falls, injury, or other safety problems.
- Ability to take prescribed drugs, or someone to supervise them.

The environment divides into the physical and social environment:
- Sufficient human help—full-time, if help may be required urgently or unpredictably; otherwise sufficient to ensure:
  - toileting
  - pressure area care
  - feeding and hygiene
  - occupation
  - social and emotional contact.
- Adequate equipment, including:
  - suitable bed and chair
  - pressure relieving mattresses and cushions
  - commode, urinals, or bedpan
  - feeding equipment (e.g. feeding pumps for PEG feeds)
  - pendant alarm or mobile phone if left alone for periods of time
  - means of entry for care staff if living alone (key safe or door entry system)
  - mobility aids (wheelchair, sticks, frame; rotunda, sliding board, or hoist for transfers)
  - rails to facilitate bed and toilet transfers.

Exceptions:
- In some cases, such as discharge for home terminal care, safety (in terms of protecting life) is not a prime concern. But many of the same considerations are needed to make the discharge practical and humane.
- Hospital is not a prison. Patients cannot be detained unless they consent, or have been shown to lack capacity and remaining in hospital is in their best interests. Remember that capacity must be assumed unless it can be demonstrated otherwise.
- Health and safety legislation applies to professional and home care staff. They cannot therefore undertake tasks carrying undue risk—for example, manual transfers represent a risk of back injury, and a hoist may be required. If the patient refuses a hoist, or there is no room, in for example, a cramped bedroom, and alternative arrangements cannot be made, staff cannot be expected to undertake transfers. Other sources of risk include aggressive or disinhibited patients with cognitive impairment.

Is appropriate community support and follow-up available?

If there are unmet rehabilitation needs, and these cannot be provided outside of hospital, then offer to provide them in hospital. Otherwise community support divides into therapeutic services (trying to improve function), and prosthetic services (making up for things the person cannot do themselves).

Therapeutic services include:
• Early discharge support and rehabilitation teams.
• Longer-term stroke disability support and rehabilitation services.
• Day hospitals.
• Generic community services such as family doctors, district nursing, community physiotherapy, social services OT (who are responsible for providing many aids and home adaptations), and speech and language therapy.
• Newer models of 'intermediate care', based in residential or nursing homes. Care must be taken to ensure that these are genuinely specialist stroke rehabilitation services, not just a convenient way of freeing up hospital beds. These services will often have scant medical and nursing staffing, and should be considered the equivalent of 'home' discharges.

Prosthetic services include:
• Social services home care, including help to get up and put to bed, washing and dressing, get meals, empty catheter bags or commodes, supervise medication, housework, and shopping.
• Meals at home service (from social services, or private equivalents, or someone to buy 'ready meals' at the supermarket and a microwave to heat them in).
• Day centres.
• Visitor and advocate schemes.
• Sitting services for carers.
• Respite care in residential or nursing homes.
• Permanent placement in a residential or nursing home.

Are the carers prepared?

The presence of a willing carer can enable a discharge that would other-wise be impossible. Such carers:

- Provide hands-on care, in much the same way as social services home care—transferring, toileting, catheter care and changing pads, getting meals, other domestic tasks, operating feeding pumps for PEG tubes, giving medication.
- Providing supervision and surveillance, looking out for problems.
- Providing company, occupation and emotional support.

The commitment of some carers, and the range of tasks they will take on is sometimes staggering. Many of these are tasks that previous everyday life has not prepared them for, such as:

- Catheter and PEG tube care.
- Safe transfers (safe for both patient and carer), or operating a hoist.
- Supervised walking.
- Dressing, and the tricks required to dress a hemiplegic person successfully (paralysed side on first and off last).
- Feeding, sometimes in patients with precarious swallowing, who need advice on positioning, consistencies, and pacing of feeds.
- Pressure area care, including turning, and operating pressure relieving mattresses.
- Administration of medicines, including insulin.
- Intermittent urinary catheterization.

These needs should be anticipated during rehabilitation, and carers given appropriate training, by OT, physiotherapy, and nursing staff.

Elderly spouses are sometimes frail themselves. Statutory services may be required to support an 'informal' carer:

- In the UK they have a statutory right to have their own needs assessed by social services departments.
- Respite care (a period in a residential or nursing home, or sometimes a hospital, to give carers a holiday or break) may need to be anticipated and arranged.
- Sitting services can allow a carer a few hours to go shopping, or to pursue social or leisure activities of their own. Opportunities for these can become very limited when caring for a very dependent person.

Is the environment optimized?

Environments can facilitate activity and participation, or provide a barrier to it. Examples include access ramps, stair rails or stair lifts, grab rails around toilets and baths, bathing equipment such as bath boards, 'glide about' chairs (with wheels on) for use in a shower, or 'bed leavers' (a rail by the bed supported under the mattress).

Wheelchair users will need sufficient space to manoeuvre, doors that are wide enough to get through and toilets with enough space to allow safe transfers. Kitchen work surfaces may need to be lower to allow use.

Home visits by OTs, with or without the patient, a physiotherapist, members of the patient's family and representatives of social services are immensely useful, and serve several purposes:

• An assessment of the physical environment, to look for hazards and other barriers.
• To plan therapeutic changes to the environment (ramps and rails, replacing or altering beds and chairs, recommending improved lighting, removal of clutter, loose wires and rugs, acquiring kitchen aids).
• Assessing the patient's performance of tasks in the home environment.
• Assessing the viability of community rehabilitation.
• To motivate and encourage the patient, as a clear indication that progress is being made, and discharge planning is taking place.
• To boost the confidence of patient and family or other carers, not least to show that proper planning is taking place.
• To demonstrate that someone will not manage at home, especially if there is dispute about this (while realizing safety is a relative and graded phenomenon, not absolute, and that a single home visit will never give a definitive assessment).

Alternative assessment opportunities include:
• Trial periods in a 'rehabilitation flat' attached to a rehabilitation unit. This can be alone, or with a carer such as a spouse. Routine professional input is limited to what a home-care package might provide.
• Overnight stay at home.
• 'Weekend leave' (i.e. several nights).

These can be used to provide information (will it work?) and to boost confidence.

Institutional discharge

The ultimate in 'environmental modification' is to abandon the previous home environment altogether, and discharge to a residential or nursing home. As a general rule, rehabilitation tries hard to avoid (or defer) this.

Residential homes were originally modelled (in the 1940s) on seaside hotels (to which elderly people would retire). The current definition is that they provide 'board, lodging, and personal care'. However, typically the prevalence of incontinence, dementia, and impaired mobility in these homes is about a third each, indicating substantial nursing and medical needs. Many residents will have developed these conditions since being admitted.

Nursing homes have at least one qualified nurse on duty all the time.

Many homes are 'dual registered' as both residential and nursing homes, and in the UK the distinction between the two is fast becoming blurred, a process largely driven by local authority payers keen to reduce costs.

With sufficient resources, it should theoretically be possible to discharge anyone home. Often institutional discharge is required when disabilities are such that adequate care cannot be provided at home within the budget available. Dementia leading to lack of judgement and safety awareness is often the deciding factor. Onset of faecal incontinence is another particular problem at home. Sometimes people decide that living at home is too dangerous or lonely. Confidence may be lost, especially if a trial of discharge ends in a fall or inability to cope. Where health has been failing for some time before the stroke, institutional care may have been contemplated prior to the stroke. Sometimes relatives push hard for institutional discharge. They will often be influential with patients, but ultimately a patient with capacity has to decide for themselves what they want, and staff should support them in this.

Sometimes people become dead-set on entry to a residential home, when the assessment of professional staff is that they could be managed at home. If the patient is paying for the care themselves, there is nothing to stop them living where they want to. But for people without means, whose care would be funded by Social Services departments, they would be assessed against eligibility criteria, and those assessed as suitable for home care may not be funded.

There can be a major problem in finding somewhere for a severely disabled younger person to live. If home discharge is impossible, there are a few nursing and residential homes specializing in the care of younger people, NHS younger disabled units, and some charities (such as the Cheshire Homes) may help.

Is there a need for follow-up?

Follow-up may be:

- Medical, to check on risk factors and secondary prevention, to follow-up the results of tests, or to check residual disability or mood.
- One of the therapies, for ongoing rehabilitation needs. A 'need' for health care implies the capacity to benefit from an intervention. This implies that someone has ongoing problems, have not reached a 'plateau', and wants to continue therapy. This may be provided in a day hospital, out-patient, or home setting.
- Supportive—such as provided by dysphasia support groups.
- To reassess for ongoing or new disabilities, problems, or mood disorders.
- Generic—patients will continue to have access to primary healthcare teams, who may refer back to specialist services if required.

Capacity and consent

Sometimes people insist on going home when rehabilitation staff are sure that they will not cope. This is usually in the context of dementia, but may occur in anosognosia (specific denial of stroke) and some other mental illnesses:

- If the patient has mental capacity to give or withhold consent, there is no question. You make things as safe as possible, in terms of environmental modification and prosthetic care, and do as the patient asks.
- If capacity is lacking, you must act in the patient's best interest. Assessing capacity and best interest in these situations can be difficult. We should assume that a patient *has* capacity, *unless* we can show that they do not. The least restrictive approach is to allow the patient to try at home—once at least.
- A second opinion (usually from a psychiatrist) is a sensible safeguard of the patient's rights (you are either considering detaining them against their will, or letting themselves be exposed to undue risk of injury).
- The views of relatives should be sought, especially as they may be required to provide a lot of the ongoing care. They may be as exasperated and helpless as you are. People with dementia are not often amenable to reasoned arguments, although some can be persuaded to have a 'trial' in a residential home. Economy with the truth is a necessary evil here—usually these are people who have settled well into the institutional hospital environment, and would likely be equally happy in a residential home.
- If a trial at home fails, and the patient is still insistent that they want to go home, you can argue that they have demonstrated sufficient lack of insight and judgement to show that they do not appreciate the consequences of their request, and therefore lack capacity. These cases can become quite intractable. You may agree to another trial at home, especially if the circumstances of the previous failure are unlikely to recur.
- There will come a stage, however, sometimes even without a first trial at home, where it is simply irresponsible to allow someone to put themselves in a position of physical danger (falling, wandering, kettles, gas, and fires), and you have to say 'no'.
- Guardianship (a legal device) is sometimes sought in these circumstances. You will need the opinion of a psychiatrist, and an approved psychiatric social worker to apply for it. Guardianship allows the guardian to specify where someone shall live, but gives no powers to enforce it (so if you can carry it out you probably didn't need it in the first place).
- The law on consent in this area is very vague. 'Persuasion' and not a little subterfuge are the mainstays of engineering what most objective observers would agree is a sensible solution. These matters cannot be taken lightly in a free country.
- We are unaware of anyone ever having been sued for irresponsibly discharging a patient who has requested it. The Courts are very supportive of professional staff acting reasonably in good faith.

Communicating with primary care: discharge summaries

Hospital doctors should communicate the details of an episode of hospital care to GPs. This also forms the definitive hospital record of the episode.

If a discharge is particularly difficult or contentious, telephone the GP in advance:

- To warn them in case something goes wrong quickly.
- They may want to visit the patient, especially if he or she is dying.
- If you want them to do something.

To be really useful a discharge summary should:

- Be typed, and confined to one side of A4 paper.
- Should reach the GP within a week of discharge (that's what GPs say they need).
- Arrive electronically, to allow uploading to their computer systems.
- Include details of the date of admissions and discharge, which wards were used and which consultants were responsible.
- The diagnosis responsible for the current admission (but remember not all GPs will know all the fashionable hospital abbreviations, so spell them out).
- All other active or relevant previous diagnoses.
- A description of the problem leading to admission, a brief history of the problem, relevant risk factors, relevant previous functional and social circumstances.
- Relevant physical signs. Include sufficient neurological details to substantiate the (Bamford) stroke syndrome diagnosed, an MMSE if done, and details of the ward BP record (a better indication of 'usual' BP than most one-off, 'casual', BP readings).
- Important investigations. Summarize (e.g. 'liver function normal'), but include information relevant to making the diagnosis (CT or MRI result), and secondary prevention (carotid duplex, ECG, echocardiograph, cholesterol).
- A summary of treatment and progress, including complications, and failed treatments (intolerance of drugs, measures for restoring continence or controlling pain), functional abilities prior to discharge, and discharge arrangements. If drugs were stopped, say so and why.
- Management plan and follow-up arrangements.
- Drugs on discharge.

Difficulties arise when the 'episode' is incomplete, and follow-up rehabilitation is occurring elsewhere, especially community services and day hospitals, and the hospital notes follow the patient to the new service. In these cases try to do the discharge summary on the day of discharge. Copy the discharge summary to involved health agencies (such as community rehabilitation), and remember that if the patient is discharged to institutional care they may change their GP.

Other primary care agencies (e.g. district nursing) also require hand-over information where they are to be involved. Information is required on mobility, continence, ADL, wound care and dressings, specific medication problems (such as anticipated compliance problems, or arrangements for drawing-up insulin injections), living arrangements, and other support services involved. GPs often find this information useful as well.

Electronic Patient Records (for hospital), Electronic Health Records (for the whole health system), and unified health and social care records ('Single Assessment Process') may alter the details of how the discharge summary is done, but the information contained will need to be the same.

Summary

1. The time for hospital discharge is when what is needed can be provided elsewhere. Hospital stay has to be well justified.
2. Much nursing and rehabilitation can be delivered at home if (and only if) there are suitable services set up locally.
3. There is no such thing as a safe discharge. There is always a degree of risk. To minimize risk requires that the patient is medically stable, has minimum levels of ability covering mobility, safety awareness, and plans for toileting or containment of incontinence, and necessary equipment, human help and environmental modifications arranged.
4. Home assessment visits are very useful, but are labour intensive and time consuming.
5. Appropriate follow-up and community support must be arranged. The term 'discharge' is sometimes frowned upon, 'transfer of care' being preferred, as it conveys a suitable concern for continuity. Carers must be prepared.
6. Where capacity to decide is lacking, and the patient wants to try a discharge which is considered high risk, you must assess best interests, but may have to go along with it at least once. Some attempts at discharge are so risky as to be irresponsible.
7. Communicate rapidly and comprehensively with primary healthcare teams.

Chapter 10

Preventing strokes and other vascular events

Vascular risks

- One in five strokes is a recurrent stroke.
- Someone who has had a first stroke is at 10-fold increased risk of another.
- Secondary prevention attempts to reduce the risk of recurrence.
- People with ischaemic heart disease and peripheral vascular disease are more likely to have a stroke, and those who have had a stroke have an increased risk of heart attack. It makes sense to consider 'vascular prevention' all together. The interventions are nearly identical in any case.

The distinction between primary and secondary prevention has been mostly abandoned in recent years. Think of it this way:

- A preventative treatment reduces risk by a certain proportion, on average (1-RR on treatment).
- How much benefit each individual gets, depends on their chances of having a vascular event at baseline (off treatment):

     absolute risk reduction = baseline risk × (1-RR on treatment).

- Baseline risk is determined by previous events, age, sex, and other risk factors such as BP, smoking, and diabetes.

We also know that:

- Most risk factors are not just present or absent, but the amount risk increases with the amount of exposure (BP, cholesterol, number of cigarettes smoked per day, blood glucose, body mass index, serum homocysteine).
- A lot of risk factors are related to each other (BP is affected by body mass index, diet, alcohol consumption, and physical activity), and some cluster together (e.g. people with diabetes often have raised BP and cholesterol).

The effects of risk factors combine together to give an overall risk:

- The Framingham risk equations (Appendices 13 and 14) enable you to put some numbers on the risk.
- Depending on how much effort and expense (money, inconvenience, side-effects) you are willing to commit to prevention (as individuals and as a society), a risk of 15–30% over 10 years is worth intervention. This is not a matter of rationing. Fifteen per cent risk over 10 years is a *low risk for the individual concerned*, for someone being asked to change life-style, or take several drugs a day for all that time.
- If someone has symptomatic vascular disease (diagnosed stroke, ischaemic heart disease, or peripheral vascular disease), their future risk almost invariably puts them in the group where prevention is justified. Most middle-aged or elderly diabetics are as well.
- Risk scores are inevitably crude, and will not include some important risk factors (or diagnoses), which are too rare to have much of an impact on population risk.

Vascular prevention (Table 10.1)

Interventions to reduce risk divide between:
- General vascular prevention (in common with ischaemic heart disease and peripheral vascular disease)
  - antithrombotics
  - BP reduction
  - cholesterol reduction
  - smoking cessation
  - other life-style interventions.
- Stroke-specific interventions:
  - carotid endarterectomy for severe stenosis
  - warfarin in atrial fibrillation.

Table 10.1 Summary of interventions to prevent stroke

Risk factor	Intervention	Evidence	Approximate RR on treatment
Life-style factors			
Smoking	Stopping	Cohort studies	0.5 after 2 years
Inactivity	Moderate exercise	Cohort studies	0.5–0.7 in various studies
Salt intake	Reduction	Systematic review of RCTs, BP end-point	0.75 per 50 mmol Na/day
Obesity	Weight loss	Cohort studies	0.5 per 6 kg/m²
Drug interventions			
BP	Drugs	Systematic reviews of RCTs	0.6 per 5–6 mmHg diastolic fall
Isolated systolic hypertension	Drugs	RCT	0.6 for 12 mmHg systolic fall
Cholesterol	Statins	Systematic reviews of RCTs	0.75 (any vascular event)
Atrial fibrillation	Warfarin (INR 2–3)	Systematic reviews of RCTs	0.3
Atrial fibrillation	Aspirin	Systematic reviews of RCTs	0.8
TIA/minor stroke	Aspirin	Systematic reviews of RCTs	0.75
Post-MI	Warfarin	Systematic reviews of RCTs	0.5
Surgical interventions			
Symptomatic carotid stenosis (70–99%)	Surgery (vs. medical)	RCT	0.5 (after 5 years inc. surgical mortality/morbidity)*
Asymptomatic carotid stenosis (60–99%)	Surgery (vs. medical)	RCT	0.5 (after 5 years inc. surgical mortality/morbidity)*

* The effect of these interventions cannot be described by a single RR. Surgical morbidity produces an immediate hazard after which strokes accumulate more slowly in surgical patients.

Box 10.1 Understanding trials in vascular prevention

Why randomized trials?

- Trials aim to establish a causal association between a treatment and an outcome.
- Random allocation aims to ensure that comparison groups are alike in all respects apart from the trial treatment they receive—i.e. the comparison is free from 'bias' and 'confounding'.

The results of a trial

- The main result is the size of the difference in outcomes between the treatments. This can be: the absolute difference in proportions experiencing an outcome (e.g. death, stroke, any cardiovascular event); or the RR of an outcome (also called the risk ratio, rate ratio, odds ratio, or hazard ratio depending on how the calculations were done).
- RR reduction is often quoted. This is (1–RR), expressed as a percentage. This number usually looks more impressive than the absolute risk difference or the RR!
- The P-value does not tell you anything about the size of the effect of treatment.
- The NNT is the number of people who must be given a treatment for 1 year to prevent one event (or cause one adverse event). It may be quoted over 5 or 10 years, in which case the NNT is five or 10 times less.
- NNT is (1/absolute risk difference) given the baseline risk in the population you are interested in. This can be estimated as 1/(estimated baseline risk × RR reduction).

Why do trials need to be big?

- Trials must be large enough to be able to measure small differences, e.g. in the Heart Protection Study all-cause mortality was reduced from 14.7% to 12.9%.
- The larger the trial, the less likely that measured differences are of the size that might also have occurred by chance. This is called the power of the trial.
- The power of the trial actually depends on the number of outcome events. A smaller trial of high-risk patients may be more powerful than a large trial of low-risk patients. To maximize power a 'combined vascular end-point' is often used (e.g. fatal and non-fatal heart attack and stroke, vascular deaths, revascularizations, and vascular amputations). This is reasonable, but look to see which components are actually showing differences as well.

P-values

- The probability that an observed difference could have arisen by chance is the P-value.
- A non-significant P-value does not mean that there is no difference. Always look at the 95% CIs for the difference between treatment arms (or the RR). This is to see how big or small the real difference could be.

- A significant *P*-value in a large trial does not tell you whether the size of the effect is of any clinical importance or not.

Intention-to-treat analysis

- A trial will underestimate the true effect of a treatment ('null bias') because of drop-outs and cross-overs (some placebo-assigned patients will get the treatment outside the trial, some active treatment-assigned patients will stop taking it).
- Trials are analysed according to ITT not 'treatment received'. This means that a placebo-assigned patient will be analysed as if they did not get the treatment, even if they receive the treatment outside the trial. Treatment-assigned subjects are analysed as if they received treatment, even if they never took it.
- The reason for ITT is to minimize the possibility of bias. People who drop out or cross-over are not representative of the group as a whole. For example, in a BP trial the placebo-assigned patients who are given active treatment outside the trial are likely to be those with the highest BPs, who are also the most likely to have a stroke. You cannot identify the patients in the active treatment group who 'match' these cross-over patients. They remain included in the treatment arm. If you exclude cross-over patients, or worse still, reassign them to the active treatment arm, you are no longer comparing like with like in terms of initial risk. The final comparison will be biased (in this example, against demonstrating an effect of the active treatment).
- An 'on treatment analysis' will often overestimate the effect of the treatment, and is only useful if you are trying to demonstrate it has no effect. In all other cases disregard such results.
- ITT to some extent replicates clinical practice when compliance is uncertain. However, this is not the main reason for doing ITT analyses.

Indirect comparisons of trial results

- The size of effect seen in any one trial will vary by chance. Indirect comparisons of different agents will often be made (especially by drug companies whose drug appears to be better), but these can be misleading.
- The best way to tell if any one treatment is really different from similar treatments is to look for a statistical test for heterogeneity in a meta-analysis of several treatment trials.
- Head-to-head comparisons of active agents are more reliable, but are fairly rare, as they need to be very large to show differences.

Practical issues

- Comparison of different agents in BP trials is complicated by the need to tailor regimens according to co-indications and adverse effects, and use drugs in combination to get adequate response.

Antithrombotics

- Aspirin reduces (ischaemic) vascular risk by about 25%. The evidence for giving 75 mg of aspirin is as strong as for any other dose, any other drug, or combination of drugs (Box 10.2).
- 75 mg of aspirin doubles the risk of peptic ulcer disease complications (bleeding, perforation). The incidence of side-effects increases rapidly with higher doses.
- Clopidogrel is very expensive. Use it in cases of true aspirin intolerance (allergy, aspirin-induced asthma, or intractable dyspepsia despite co-administration of a proton pump inhibitor). Dipyridamole (modified release 200 mg bd) is an acceptable alternative.
- 'Aspirin failure' does not exist. All preventative treatments reduce, not eliminate, the risk of further events. Adding clopidogrel to aspirin produces no net benefit.
- One large trial (ESPS-2) suggested additional benefit for aspirin plus dipyridamole over aspirin alone. This result was not consistent other evidence in systematic reviews, and may have been due to a chance larger-than-average effect for dipyridamole combined with a smaller-than-expected effect for aspirin (in a dose of 50 mg/day).
- Warfarin (INR 3–4) in the absence of atrial fibrillation causes more intracerebral bleeds than it prevents infarcts.
- For patients with very frequent recurrences, sometimes a combination of aspirin and warfarin is used. This is an unproven strategy. Make sure that the diagnosis is right (fits or migraine can deceive even experienced doctors).
- Co-prescribe a proton pump inhibitor in high-risk groups (history of peptic ulcer in the past 10 years, co-prescription of corticosteroids or non-steroidal anti-inflammatory drugs). Ibuprofen may diminish the protective effect of aspirin.
- If a patients develops anaemia on aspirin, investigate it (haematinics, upper gastrointestinal endoscopy, and large bowel investigations if necessary and appropriate).

Box 10.2 Antiplatelet agents prevent strokes and other vascular events: Anti-Thrombotic Trialists collaboration

- The collaboration included 197 trials of antiplatelet therapy vs. control ($n = 136\,000$), 90 comparisons of different antiplatelet regimens ($n = 77\,000$), and 17 000 outcome vascular events (MI, stroke, or vascular death), including 4900 strokes.
- Aspirin reduced vascular events with an RR on treatment of 0.75 (95% CI 0.71–0.79), for patients at high risk of vascular disease (>3%/year). Vascular death (RR 0.85, 95% CI 0.81–0.89), and all-cause mortality were reduced.
- Aspirin reduced non-fatal strokes (RR 0.75, 95% CI 0.69–0.81), with no difference between categories of patient treated (prior MI, acute MI, prior stroke or TIA, other high risk).
- Overall RR of any stroke on treatment was 0.78 (95% CI 0.72–0.84). Haemorrhagic strokes increased on treatment (RR 1.22, 95% CI 1.03–1.44), but ischaemic strokes decreased (RR 0.70, 95% CI 0.65–0.76).
- Greater case fatality in haemorrhagic strokes offset the reduction in fatal strokes (RR 0.84, 95% CI 0.70–0.98).
- Disabling strokes and fatal strokes together were reduced (RR 0.76, 95% CI 0.58–0.94).
- Aspirin reduced total vascular events among 18 000 patients with a prior history of stroke or TIA (RR 0.78, 95% CI 0.70–0.86). Patients with TIA and completed strokes had the same benefit.
- The effect was regardless of aspirin dose (down to 75 mg/day).
- Doses below 75 mg/day may be less effective than 75–150 mg/day, but with current data differences are within the range that might have been expected by chance.
- Benefit continued to be observed into the second and third years of treatment.
- 787 major extracranial bleeds were recorded, RR on treatment 1.6 (95% CI 1.4–1.8).
- Clopidogrel reduced vascular events slightly more than aspirin (RR 0.91, 95% CI 0.83–0.99).
- There was no definite additional benefit from adding dipyridamole to aspirin. RR on combination therapy (for total vascular events) in direct comparisons vs. aspirin alone was 0.94 (95% CI 0.82–1.06). RR for combination therapy vs. placebo was 0.70 (95% CI 0.62–0.78), compared with 0.77 (0.73–0.81) for aspirin at any dose vs. placebo, or 0.68 (0.56–0.80) for 75–150 mg aspirin vs. placebo.
- Healthy people at low risk of vascular events (<1% per year) did not benefit from aspirin.

British Medical Journal 1994; **308**: 81–106, and 2002; **324**: 71–86

Smoking

- Smoking doubles the risk of both cerebral infarcts and bleeds.
- Risk reduces to near that of never-smokers within 2 years of stopping.
- It is never too late to give up.
- Professional or group support, nicotine replacement, and bupropion all increase the chances of successfully quitting (5% give up on advice alone, 10–20% with drug treatment).
- Many patients successfully use the opportunity of hospitalization for stroke to stop. Discuss and encourage this.
- Stopping smoking is hard, and may take several attempts. Relapse is common. Sympathize, don't blame or stigmatize.
- Withdrawal symptoms include craving, inability to concentrate, irritability, and general malaise.
- The more times you try stopping, the better your chances of ultimate success!

Blood pressure

Principles

- BP is causally related to risk of stroke.
- Risk increases 40% for each 10 mmHg increase in systolic BP. For stroke, this risk is reversed within a few years of treatment. For ischaemic heart disease about half the increased risk is reversed within a few years.
- Reduction of BP is important above all else, regardless of which drugs are used (Boxes 10.3 and 10.4).
- Isolated systolic hypertension is as important as combined systolic and diastolic hypertension.
- BP is often raised after a stroke, and will reduce spontaneously over about a week. For secondary prevention start (or increase) drugs after that.
- Do not treat a single, one-off, BP reading. Clinic readings are often raised. Five minutes of lying down, followed by a nurse-measured BP, is often better. A ward observations record is a good guide to 'usual' BP. If in doubt about degree of hypertension, or 'white coat' hypertension, get 24-h ambulatory monitoring.
- The lower the BP the better, so long as symptomatic hypotension is not induced (postural dizziness or syncope, mainly). Less than 140/85 is a reasonable target and audit standard. Less than 130/80 is suggested for diabetics—ideally this should go for anyone with a stroke as well.
- For a preventative intervention, troublesome side-effects of treatment are not to be tolerated (you should not sacrifice current well-being for uncertain future benefits).
- BP control will usually be monitored in primary care. Those who can afford it might be encouraged to buy a home BP monitoring machine (about £80 in the UK; search the internet or ask at a pharmacy).
- BP is usually undertreated in the UK.
- Monotherapy is unlikely to be effective—there are multiple physiological BP control systems, and inhibiting one will often produce counter-regulation in others.
- Use effective doses.

Which drugs?

- Stroke patients often have other things wrong with them, and antihypertensive therapy can be tailored to take into account additional benefits, and to avoid particular side-effects or complications (Table 10.2).
- Thiazides (bendroflumethazide/bendrofluazide 2.5 mg daily) are the best established antihypertensives, are cheap, and in comparative studies have equal (or better) efficacy, and the same incidence of side-effects as any other agents (Box 10.3).
- ACEI have a good track record in vascular secondary prevention (Boxes 10.5 and 10.6):
  - They are useful when there is comorbid heart or renal failure, diabetes, or previous MI.

- A proportion of stroke patients will also have renovascular disease. Check biochemical renal function, and recheck a fortnight after starting. If BP is difficult to control, get renal artery Doppler studies or a magnetic resonance angiogram.
- The action is probably a class effect. Enalapril, lisinopril, ramipril, and perindopril all have hard end-point (total vascular events) trials supporting their use. Enalapril is the cheapest. Perindopril has the advantage of rapid titration up to its maximum dose.
- Some evidence suggests an effect of ACEIs/angiotensin receptor blockers beyond that explained by BP reduction, but this has yet to be consistently born out in large trials.
- BP in Afro-Caribbean and elderly people is less responsive to manipulation of the renin–angiotensin system.
- Angiotensin II receptor inhibitors seem to have all the benefits of ACEIs, and avoid the problem of ACEI-induced cough.
- CCBs are safe and effective. But they can cause troublesome oedema and constipation. The ALLHAT trial (Box 10.3) suggested an increase in heart failure compared with thiazides.
- Alpha-blockers are useful when there is bladder outflow obstruction due to benign prostatic hyperplasia (terazosin or doxazosin), or incomplete bladder emptying poststroke. However, in the biggest comparative trial, treatment based on doxazosin prevented fewer cardiovascular events, especially heart failure and stroke, than did treatment based on chlorthalidone (Box 10.3).
- Beta-blockers are useful if there is also ischaemic heart disease or heart failure. In a number of trials atenolol has performed marginally less well than its comparators (e.g. thiazides, losartan), but we lack a large definitive trial.
- Two-thirds of patients will need more than one drug to get adequate control. The British Hypertension Society recommend a five stage approach, with some combinations pharmacologically more logical than others (Table 10.3). There is a growing case for using combination products to simplify drug regimens and reduce the numbers of tablets taken, although these have been frowned upon in the past.

Table 10.2 Co-indications, benefits, and common adverse effects of antihypertensive drugs

Drug	Useful co-indications and other benefits	Common adverse effects
Thiazides	Less heart failure, can reduce nocturnal polyuria, cheap	Hypokalaemia, hyponatraemia, gout, impotence, glucose intolerance, or diabetes. Generally don't co-prescribe with loop diuretics
Beta-blockers	Angina, post-MI, heart failure, tachyarrhythmias, anxiety, migraine, cheap	Cold peripheries, fatigue, wheeze, impotence, heart block, heart failure, sleep disturbance, nightmares
CCBs	Angina, tachyarrhythmias	Oedema, constipation, heart failure, headache
ACEIs	Heart failure, post-MI, diabetes, renal failure	Cough, renal failure, angio-oedema, hypotension, especially if dehydrated or aortic stenosis
Alpha-blockers	Prostatic hyperplasia, incomplete bladder emptying	First dose hypotension, lethargy, rhinitis, stress incontinence in women
Spironolactone	Heart failure	Nausea, diarrhoea, impotence, hyperkalaemia
Angiotensin II receptor antagonists (ARB)	Heart failure	Few side-effects, expensive

Table 10.3 British Hypertension Society guidelines on drug combinations

Step		Drug
1	Age under 55 years	ACEI/ARB (A) or beta-blocker (B)
	Black or age over 55	Thiazide (D) or CCB (C)
2		A or B add D or C
3		A, C, D
4		A, C, D, add alpha-blocker
5		A, C, D, alpha-blocker, add spironolactone

http://www.bhsoc.org

Box 10.3 ALLHAT (Antihypertensive and Lipid Lowering to prevent Heart Attack Trial): BP lowering based on different classes of drugs was about equally effective

- The study compared antihypertensive treatment regimens based on chlorthalidone (a thiazide diuretic, 12.5–25 mg/day, the 'standard' comparator), amlodipine (2.5–10 mg/day, a CCB), lisinopril (10–40 mg/day, an ACEI), and doxazosin (2–8 mg/day, an alpha blocker).
- To avoid 'contamination' between groups recommended add-on drugs for inadequate control included atenolol, reserpine, and hydralazine.
- 42 424 patients, over 55 years old, with BP above 140/90, and with at least one other cardiovascular risk factor were randomized—90% were switched from other hypertensive treatments for the trial.
- BP control was less good in the lisinopril group (2 mmHg systolic).
- 80% of the chlorthalidone and amlodipine group were receiving the study drug or another of the same class after 5 years, as were 70% of the lisinopril patients.
- The doxazosin arm was terminated early after median follow-up of 3.3 years. Compared with chlorthalidone there was no difference in the primary outcome (MI plus vascular deaths, RR 1.03, 95% CI 0.90–1.17), or all-cause mortality (RR 1.03, 95% CI 0.90–1.15). However, doxazosin-treated patients had more strokes (RR 1.19, 1.01–1.40), total vascular events (25% vs. 22%, RR 1.25, 1.17–1.33), and heart failure (RR 2.04, 1.79–2.32).
- The other comparisons had mean follow-up of 4.9 years. The primary outcome occurred in 11.3–11.5%, with no differences between groups (RR 0.98–0.99, 95% CI ± 0.10). All-cause mortality did not differ. Amlodipine treatment was associated with more heart failure (RR1.38, 95% CI 1.25–1.52), and lisinopril treatment was associated with more total vascular events (RR 1.10, 95% CI 1.05–1.15), stroke (RR 1.15, 95% CI 1.02–1.30), and heart failure (RR 1.19, 95% CI 1.07–1.31).
- This trial supports the need to reduce BP using whichever drug classes are required to do so. Excess heart failure in the amlodipine group could be due to the diuretic effect of thiazides, or the negative inotropic effect of amlodipine. The excess strokes in the lisinopril group may have been due to less good BP control.

JAMA 2000; **283**: 1967–75
JAMA 2002; **288**: 2981–97

Box 10.4 Are some antihypertensive drugs more effective than others?

- Nine BP reduction trials in 62 605 hypertensive patients without heart failure were included in a meta-analysis. Older drugs (diuretics and beta-blockers) were compared with newer classes (CCBs, ACEIs, and alpha-blockers).
- The relationship between risk reduction, BP difference between arms of the trial, and baseline BP was also studied with data from 136 124 patients in 27 trials.
- The outcome was combined fatal and non-fatal vascular events, with mean follow-up of 2–8 years.
- ACEIs and CCBs were as effective, but no more so, than diuretics and beta-blockers at preventing vascular mortality, but CIs were wide, so an important effect one way or the other could have been missed (odds ratio 95% CIs 0.91–1.21 for CCBs, 0.83–1.16 for ACEIs).
- ACEIs and CCBs were slightly less effective, than diuretics and beta-blockers at preventing total vascular events (OR 95% CI 0.93–1.09 for CCB, 0.95–1.09 for ACEI). CCBs may have been more effective at preventing stroke (OR 0.87, 95% CI 0.76–0.99), offset by lesser reduction in risk of MI.
- Individual trials gave a few apparently anomalous results in particular subgroups (more fatal MI on nifedipine, more strokes on captopril, fewer strokes on diltiazem). Most likely these were chance findings, as there was no consistent or logical pattern.
- There was a linear relationship between BP differences and odds ratio for vascular mortality, and a curvilinear relationship for total vascular events and stroke. Baseline BP had little effect on risk reduction.
- Observed risk differences between drugs were no more than would be expected by chance.
- BP reduction is important regardless of the particular drugs used to achieve it. No drug or drug class was clearly superior to any other.

Lancet 2001; **358**: 1305–15

Box 10.5 PROGRESS trial: BP reduction prevents stroke recurrence

- 6105 patients who had had a non-disabling stroke or TIA were randomly assigned BP lowering treatment or placebo, regardless of whether their BP was 'high' or 'normal' (or even 'low'). No lower limit was placed on BP for entry to the trial.
- Active treatment was perindopril (ACEI) 2 mg, increasing to 4 mg after 2 weeks, with indapamide (a thiazide) 2.5 mg added at the discretion of the investigator. Combination treatment could be pre-specified, and randomization was stratified for this choice.
- BP was reduced by 9/4 mmHg on average. Follow-up was 4 years. New stroke was the primary outcome.
- Half of participants were on other BP drugs at the time of randomization. Thus, benefits of the trial treatment were additional to that gained by being on treatment already.
- RRs on treatment were:
  - 0.72 (95% CI 0.62–0.83) for any stroke (13.8% vs. 10.0%)
  - 0.96 (0.82–1.12) for all-cause mortality (10.4% vs. 10.0%)
  - 0.76 (0.72–0.81) for any major vascular event (15.0% vs. 19.8%)
- RRs on treatment were greater on combination therapy (mean BP reduction 12/5 mmHg) compared with single drug (mean BP reduction 5/3 mmHg).
  - for stroke: 0.95 (0.77–1.19, i.e. no effect) single drug vs. 0.57 (0.46–0.70) combined
  - for major vascular events: 0.96 (0.80–1.15) single drug vs. 0.60 (0.51–0.71) combined
- Reduced risk on treatment was similar regardless of type of stroke, and initial BP (i.e. reducing 'normal' BP is beneficial).

Lancet 2001; **358**: 1033–41

Box 10.6 Heart Outcome Prevention Evaluation (HOPE) study

- Tested the effect of ACEI ramipril in people with high vascular risk but without left ventricular dysfunction or heart failure.
- 9297 patients over 55 years old with vascular disease or diabetes plus one other vascular risk factor, randomized to 10 mg ramipril or placebo for a mean 5 years.
- 11% of participants had stroke, 80% ischaemic heart disease, and 40% peripheral vascular disease. Half were diagnosed hypertensive, and 40% were diabetic. Most were on other vascular preventative treatments.
- A run-in phase excluded about 10% of potential patients because of non-compliance, side-effects, or abnormal renal function or potassium.
- Dose was escalated as 2.5 mg a day for 1 week, 5 mg a day for 3 weeks then 10 mg.
- 87% were taking ramipril or another ACEI at 1 year, 75% at 4 years—10% of the placebo group patients were receiving an ACEI at 4 years.
- Entry mean BP was 139/79. BP difference on active treatment was 4/2 at 1 month and 3/1 mmHg at the end of the study.
- RRs on treatment were:
  - 0.78 (95% CI 0.70–0.86) for any major vascular event (14.0% vs. 17.8%)
  - 0.74 (0.64–0.87) for cardiovascular deaths (6.1% vs. 8.1%)
  - 0.84 (0.75–0.95) for all-cause mortality (10.4% vs. 12.2%)
  - 0.80 (0.70–0.90) for MI (9.9% vs. 12.3%)
  - 0.68 (0.56–0.84) for stroke (3.4% vs. 4.9%)
- Benefits were seen in both sexes, in participants with and without diabetes, cardiovascular disease, stroke, and hypertension, and regardless of age and left ventricle ejection fraction.
- When this study was performed, benefits of ACEIs had been established in patients with heart failure, left ventricular dysfunction, and after heart attack. This study demonstrated a benefit on the basis of high baseline risk, and irrespective of baseline BP. BP reduction with treatment was small. The investigators speculated that there might have been an additional non-BP benefit.
- A subsequent study (EUROPA) showed similar effects for 8 mg/day perindopril in lower risk patients with stable ischaemic heart disease.

New England Journal of Medicine 2000; **342**: 145–53
British Medicine Journal 2002; **324**: 699–702
Lancet 2003; **362**: 782–8

Cholesterol

- For many years it appeared that cholesterol concentration was not a risk factor for stroke. This was possibly because of inability to separate ischaemic stroke (risk increases with higher cholesterol) from haemorrhagic stroke (risk decreases with higher cholesterol) in older studies.

- In prevention trials of statins for people with ischaemic heart disease, incidence of stroke was reduced by 31% (as well as the benefits in preventing other vascular disease).

- The Heart Protection Study treated all patients (with simvastatin 40 mg or placebo) deemed at high risk, by virtue of a previous vascular event, diabetes or multiple vascular risk factors, and regardless of their initial cholesterol. There was a 25% reduction in vascular events, including in the patients who had had a previous stroke (Box 10.7).

- Outside of specialized lipid clinic practice, HMG CoA reductase inhibitors (statins) are the only useful drugs. Dietary advice is wise (weight loss, low animal fat, functional foods, e.g. Benecol®), and effects are additional to those of drugs, but statins are considerably more powerful than the effect of diet alone.

- Simvastatin is well proven, reduces cholesterol by about 50%, and soon will be off-patent. Start at the top dose—40 mg (some doctors still titrate up in the hope of averting minor side-effects). Myositis is a rare but important complication (measure creatine kinase if worried). Rosuvastatin and atorvastatin reduce cholesterol by an additional 10% or so.

Box 10.7 Heart Protection Study (HPS)

- Participants were 20 536 people aged 40–80 years at high risk of vascular death by virtue of a prior vascular event (including 3280 who had had a stroke), diabetes, or treated hypertension in men over 65 years old, and with a total cholesterol greater than 3.5 mmol/l.
- They were given simvastatin 40 mg a day or placebo, and followed up for 5 years.
- On average 85% of the intervention group took their drug, and 17% of the control group were given an out-of-trial statin. Total cholesterol was reduced on average by 1.2 mmol/l (low-density lipoprotein cholesterol by 1.0 mmol/l), but the difference between intervention and control dropped from 1.7 mmol/l in the first year, to 0.8 mmol/l in the 5th year.
- RRs on treatment were:
  - 0.87 (95% CI 0.81–0.94) for all-cause mortality (12.9% vs. 14.7%)
  - 0.76 (0.72–0.81) for any major vascular event (19.8% vs. 25.2%)
  - 0.75 (0.66–0.85) for any stroke (and TIA) (4.3% vs. 5.7%)
- There was no increase in haemorrhagic strokes (although numbers were few and this was statistically uncertain), nor fatal or more severe strokes.
- There were no differences in effect according the presence or absence of coronary artery disease, prior disease category that allowed entry to the trial, age, sex, initial cholesterol level or any other variable, including other preventative drug treatments. This indicated that the effects are additive to those of the other treatments.
- Myositis was very rare (10 simvastatin vs. 4 placebo).

Lancet 2002; **360**: 7–22

Life-style changes

- The evidence for the effectiveness of interventions to promote life-style changes is poor (Box 10.8).
- Effects often wane over a year or so—advice will need repeating.
- Changes may help promote a sense of taking control of responsibility for health. They should all be discussed with patients who survive with no more than mild to moderate disability.
- BP can be reduced by (in approximate order of efficacy):
  - weight loss
  - reducing heavy alcohol intake
  - eating more fruit and vegetables
  - restricting salt intake.
- None of these approaches the efficacy of drug treatment.
- Moderate exercise, for at least 20 min, at least three times a week, preferably daily. Try to build this into the daily routine (getting to work, work, stairs, housework, gardening, shopping).
- Weight loss probably has benefits beyond those on BP and cholesterol, and relief of stress on arthritic knees. Aim for 5–10% over 3 months. This is realistically achievable and sustainable.
- Reduce alcohol intake to standard 'sensible' limits (men <21 units/week, women <14 units/week, half this in people >75 years old, abstention for people with a history of alcohol problems; 1 unit = 10 g ethanol, 1 small glass wine, single measure spirits, half pint/250 ml beer).

Hormone replacement therapy and the contraceptive pill

- Combined oestrogen–progestogen HRT increases the risk of stroke and should be avoided unless there are troublesome menopausal symptoms (certainly after a stroke).
- The combined oral contraceptive pill also increases the RR of stroke, but the absolute risks are low in young women. If someone has a stroke on the pill, alternative contraception should be found (progesterone-only pill, IUCD, barrier methods or sterilization).

Box 10.8 Trials of life-style changes

- A 2×2 factorial trial of weight loss, dietary sodium restriction, or both, was carried out in 2382 participants with 'high normal' BP (mean 128/86) who were slightly overweight:
  - Mean weight reduction in the intervention group compared with the usual care group was 4.5 kg at 6 months, and 2 kg after 3 years.
  - Mean sodium excretion was less in the sodium reduction group compared with the usual care group, by 50 mmol/day after 6 months, and 40 mmol/day after 3 years, but only 35 mmol/day after 6 months and 25 mmol/day after 3 years in the combined group.
  - Mean BP at 6 months reduced 3.7/2.7 mmHg in the weight loss group, 2.9/1.6 mmHg in the sodium reduction group, and 4.0/2.8 mmHg in the combined group, but this waned to 1.3/0.9 mmHg after 3 years. Over 4 years there was a 20% reduction in the incidence of 'hypertension' (BP over 140/90) in both intervention groups.
- Another trial studied 201 men with high normal BP, and intervened to achieve a 2.7 kg mean weight reduction, 25% reduced mean sodium intake, and 30% decreased reported alcohol intake:
  - Mean BP reduced 2.0/1.9 mmHg. RR of developing 'hypertension' in the intervention compared with control groups was 0.42, 95% CI 0.21–0.83 (19.2% vs. 8.8%).
- A third trial randomized 459 participants between a control diet, a fruit and vegetable rich diet, and a fruit and vegetable rich, low fat diet:
  - Initial mean BP was 131/85 mmHg. The intervention diets reduced this over 8 weeks by 2.8/1.1 and 5.5/3.0 mmHg. Among hypertensive subjects mean reductions were up to 11/6 mmHg.
- Intervention entailed intensive advice and support from dieticians, doctors, psychologists, and counsellors, individually and in groups, including involvement of family members, up to weekly initially, and 1–2 monthly after that in two of the trials, and central preparation of all meals in the third trial.
- Life-style modification does reduce BP. Changes are difficult to maintain over long periods of time. BP reductions are small compared with those that can be achieved with drugs.

Archives of Internal Medicine 1997; **157**: 657–67
JAMA 1989; **262**: 1801–7
New England Journal of Medicine 1997; **336**: 1117–24

Carotid stenosis

- Patients with anterior circulation stroke, who survive with no more than mild to moderate disability, and who would be willing to have an operation, should be screened for carotid stenosis on the symptomatic side by duplex scanning, MR or CT angiography.
- Most lacunar strokes are not caused by carotid atheroma, but distinguishing them from partial anterior circulation strokes is not always reliable.
- Patients with greater than 70% stenosis benefit overall from carotid endarterectomy, so long as the surgeon has an audited average complication rate (death or disabling stroke) of <5% (Box 10.9). For every 20 operations done, one patient has a stroke perioperatively, and four patients avoid a stroke over the next 5 years. There is a 1 in 100 chance of death, and a 1 in 40 chance of a cranial nerve palsy (hoarse voice, usually recovers). These odds should be explained to the patient.
- Aim for surgery as soon as possible after minor stroke or TIA, ideally within 2 weeks.
- Carotid angioplasty and stenting is a reasonable alternative to surgical endarterectomy, where there is local neuroradiological expertise. Overall outcomes (strokes and deaths) after 3 years follow-up are about the same; cranial nerve palsies (8.7% vs. 0) and bleeding complications (7% vs. 1%) are much less; but there is a greater chance of recurrence of the stenosis than with surgery (14% vs. 4% after a year).
- Asymptomatic carotid stenosis (usually the other side when a potentially symptomatic artery is investigated) is not an indication for carotid surgery. Two trials demonstrated a reduction in stroke rate following operation (from 10% to 5% over 5 years, with a very low perioperative complication rate of 2%). The baseline risk of stroke attributable to asymptomatic stenosis is low. You need to do 100 operations to prevent one stroke in a year.

Box 10.9 Carotid surgery trials

- Two large-scale randomized trials have studied the efficacy of carotid endarterectomy in preventing strokes—the European Carotid Surgery Trial (ECST) and the North American Symptomatic Carotid Endarterectomy Trial (NASCET). Results (on 6092 patients) have been pooled and reanalysed.
- Follow-up was 1–167 months, mean 65 months, giving 35 000 person-years of follow-up, and 1265 patients experiencing a stroke or death.
- 10% were over 75 years; 43% had a stroke, 38% TIA, and 19% ocular events. All were randomized within 6 months of the qualifying event, 41% within a month.
- ECST and NASCET adopted different conventions for describing degree of internal carotid stenosis on angiograms. The reanalysis adopted the NASCET convention. NASCET 50% is ECST 65%, and NASCET 70% is ECST 82%. 'Near-occlusion' (underfilling of the distal internal carotid) was a separate category.
- Comparison was between surgery (most performed within 14 days of randomization) plus best medical management, vs. medical management alone.
- Outcomes included any stroke lasting more than 24 h. Disabling stroke was defined as a Rankin score of 3 or more (need for help from others).
- Surgery was associated with a perioperative (30 days) risk (1.1% deaths, 7.1% death or stroke). Medical management has a steady accrual of risk over time. A single RR cannot describe findings adequately.
- Absolute risk reductions with surgery, for any stroke or operative death after 5 years were:
    - –0.1% (95% CI –10% to +10%) for near occlusion (22% surgical vs. 22% medical)
    - 15% (10–21%) for 70–99% stenosis (16% vs. 31%)
    - 8% (3–13%) for 50–69% stenosis (19% vs. 27%)
    - 3% (–2 to 7%) for 30–49% stenosis (21% vs. 24%)
    - –3% (–6 to +1%) for <30% stenosis (18% vs. 15%)
- Absolute risk reductions with surgery, for disabling or fatal ipsilateral stroke after 5 years or operative stroke or death, were:
    - –2% (95% CI –9% to +4%) for near occlusion (8% surgical vs. 6% medical)
    - 7% (4–10%) for 70–99% stenosis (3% vs. 10%)
    - 2% (0–5%) for 50–69% stenosis (3% vs. 5%)
    - 0 (–2 to +3%) for 30–49% stenosis (5% vs. 5%)
    - –2% (–4 to 0%) for <30% stenosis (4% vs. 2%)
- NNT for 50–69% stenosis is 13 over 5 years, but the reduction in disabling stroke was very small. NNT is 6 for 70–99% stenosis.

Lancet 2003; **361**: 107–16

Atrial fibrillation

- Risk of stroke is increased fivefold in the presence of atrial fibrillation. Risks are higher in the presence of other risk factors, including heart failure and hypertension, and with increasing age (Box 10.10).
- Warfarin treatment reduces the risk by two-thirds, at the cost of the inconvenience of having to be monitored, about 2–4%/year chance of severe bleeding (requiring admission or transfusion), and up to 50% chance of minor bleeding per year (Box 10.11).
- Aspirin treatment is less effective, reducing strokes by one-fifth, but at considerably less risk (0.5% per year chance of gastrointestinal bleeding).
- A new (as yet unavailable) drug, ximelagatran (36 mg bd), is at least as effective as warfarin, and probably safer.
- Commence warfarin 1–2 weeks after stroke onset, after intracranial haemorrhage has been excluded by CT scanning. Aim for INR 2–3.
- Estimate absolute stroke risk for your patient (see Appendix 14). Use this to estimate the absolute risk reduction and number needed to treat. This may help in counselling and decision making about warfarin, and may aid compliance.
- Reasons for not giving warfarin include history of intracerebral bleeding, likely poor compliance or anticipated problems with monitoring, possible systemic bleeding (e.g. unexplained iron deficiency anaemia), frequent falls, and patient choice.

Other cardio-embolism

Anticoagulation with warfarin is also sensible for patients who are within 3 months of a MI, have mitral stenosis, a mechanical prosthetic heart valve, or presumed paradoxical embolism via a patent foramen ovale, and in whom it is not otherwise contra-indicated.

Box 10.10 Stroke risk in atrial fibrillation

- Pooled data from prevention trials were used to derive risk models for stroke in atrial fibrillation.
- Age, history of hypertension, and previous stroke or TIA all increased risk of stroke. Annual risks for age <65, 65–75, and >75 years with no risk factors were 1.0%, 4.3%, and 3.5%. With one or more additional risk factors, risk was 4.9%, 5.7%, and 8.1% per year.
- Another study identified heart failure, hypertension, and previous thromboembolism as risk factors. Risks were 2.5%/year if none of the factors was present, 7.2%/year for one factor, 17.6%/year for two or three factors.
- In addition echocardiographic global left ventricular dysfunction, and left atrial size >4.7 cm were independent risk factors, with annual risks for none, 1 or 2, and three or more of these factors of 1.0%, 6%, and 18.6%
- A comprehensive risk model for patients with atrial fibrillation has been developed from the Framingham study (see Appendix 14)

Archives of Internal Medicine 1994; **154**: 1449–57; *JAMA* 2003; **290**: 1049–56

Box 10.11 Anticoagulation or aspirin in patients with atrial fibrillation

- The European Atrial Fibrillation study randomized 1007 patients, with a recent stroke or TIA and atrial fibrillation, to aspirin 300 mg, warfarin anticoagulation, or placebo, and a further 2338 patients for whom anticoagulation was contraindicated, to aspirin or placebo.
- RRs on warfarin were:
  - 0.53 (95% CI 0.36–0.79) for combined vascular death, stroke, MI, or peripheral embolism (8%/year vs. 17%/year)
  - 0.82 (95% CI 0.54–1.26) for all-cause mortality (8%/year vs. 9%/year)
  - 0.34 (95% CI 0.20–0.57) for stroke (4%/year vs. 12%/year).
- There was no waning of treatment efficacy with time.
- Warfarin was more effective than aspirin (RR 0.60, 0.41–0.87, NNT 19), and aspirin was probably more effective than placebo (RR 0.83, 0.65–1.05, NNT 25).
- Major bleeds were 2.8% per year for warfarin, 0.9% per year for aspirin, and 0.7% per year for placebo.
- These RRs are similar to those from pooled data in primary prevention studies (participants with atrial fibrillation without prior stroke)
  - 0.32 (95% CI 0.21–0.50) for warfarin vs. placebo
  - 0.79 (95% CI 0.62–1.0) for aspirin (75–325 mg/day) vs. placebo.
- Overall risks for patients on warfarin were minimized at an INR of 2–3.

Lancet 1993; **342**: 1255–62; *Archives of Internal Medicine* 1994; **154**: 1449–57; *Archives of Internal Medicine* 1997; **157**: 1237–40

Pragmatics and compliance

It is not uncommon to see patients admitted to hospital taking 10 or 15 different drugs. Evidence suggests that compliance on the fourth drug is 50%. But you don't know which the fourth drug is.

Help improve compliance if you can.

- Simplify the drug regimen as far as possible:
  - be sure that each drug is necessary (diuretics, analgesics, sedatives, hypnotics, and laxatives, in particular, should be reviewed critically);
  - use once-a-day drugs or formulations whenever possible;
  - use fixed-dose combinations if these are available and suitable.
- If you stop or start drugs during a hospital admission, especially an unusual drug or one used for an unusual indication, explicitly tell the GP in the discharge summary or clinic letter, so that stopped drugs are not inadvertently restarted, or useful drugs stopped during a routine drug review.
- Know if a particular drug is prone to side-effects and find out if those effects are occurring. This is a particular issue with loop diuretics causing urinary frequency, urgency, and incontinence in older people, who then often don't take them. For most preventative treatments side-effects are unacceptable (you cause a problem now to prevent something that may never happen—and often the odds are usually that it will never happen).
- Make remembering what tablets to take when as easy to take as possible:
  - ensure patients understand their drugs, know what they are for, and when to take them—nurses and pharmacists can help here;
  - explain drug changes as you make them—some patients are bemused and upset by apparently random stopping and starting of drugs on ward rounds;
  - self-administration of drugs while in hospital helps with familiarity, gives practice, and can alert staff to patients who cannot take drugs reliably;
  - on discharge, write down what to take when;
  - use 'dosette' boxes or commercial blister pack services (from retail pharmacists—at a cost) if necessary;
  - enlist support from relatives to supervise tablet taking;
  - social services home care will often prompt to take tablets, but will not usually administer them;
  - you can assume that patients in residential or nursing homes will have medication administered reliably.
- Stroke patients may not be able to open child-resistant containers. Check, and provide alternatives if necessary.

Neurovascular or transient ischaemic attack clinics

The rate of recurrent TIA or stroke after a first TIA (or minor stroke) is 8% within a week, 12% within a month, and 17% within 3 months. A third of these are fatal or disabling. After that annual rate of stroke is 5% and MI 2.5%.

Rapid access (within days) to a clinic is an alternative to admission for investigation of TIA or minor non-disabling stroke. If this is not possible, admission for investigation is probably in the patient's best interests.

Diagnosis

The diagnosis and differential diagnoses of cerebrovascular disorders were described in Chapter 1. Confirming the diagnosis is the first function of a TIA clinic. Many non-specific or transient symptoms need an explanation. However, the following problems in isolation are not TIAs, and are best dealt with elsewhere:

- Confusion or forgetfulness
- Dizziness or light-headedness
- Blackouts or syncope
- Falls
- Incontinence
- Generalized weakness or sensory symptoms.

Neurological features, which if present in isolation, are not suggestive of TIA, include:

- Paraparesis or quadriparesis
- Visual hallucinations (might occur due to lesions in the occipital, parietal or temporal lobe, but are more commonly seen in delirium or Lewy body dementia)
- Dysarthria
- Vertigo (ischaemically induced isolated vertigo is possible but rare)
- Dysphagia
- Amnesia
- Diplopia
- Hearing loss

TIA is suggested when:

- Sudden onset, transient focal features (e.g. face or limb weakness, dysphasia, monocular blindness).
- A combination of features such as diplopia, dysarthria and dysphagia of sudden onset suggest brainstem ischaemia.

Investigations

- *Carotid duplex scanning.* TIA clinics should have immediate access to carotid duplex scanning. It is sensible to screen out people who have not had an anterior circulation TIA clinically, or had confirmed lacunar strokes or bleeds on neuroimaging, and possibly those who would not want an operation if offered it (although knowing you have a tight stenosis might be a factor in deciding). If a tight stenosis is detected, this is often followed up with MR, CT, or other angiography, to confirm the stenosis and look for distal vascular disease that might complicate or contra-indicate surgery.

- *Neuroimaging*. Imaging shows an infarct relevant to the symptoms in about 25% of people who have had a TIA. A few will have an alternative diagnosis, and very few will have small bleeds, and these may be saved further work up and possible risks of carotid endarterectomy. Clinical uncertainty will indicate a scan in others. Ideally the 'one-stop' approach should include CT scanning, but this should not be prioritized above prompt scanning for patients with established strokes. If the symptoms last less than 1 h, they can usually be assumed to be of ischaemic origin.
- *Cardiological investigations*. 12-lead ECG to diagnose atrial fibrillation, evidence of ischaemic heart disease, and left ventricular hypertrophy. Follow this up with echocardiography if there is a history of cardiac disease or reason to suspect cardio-embolism.

Management of transient ischaemic attack

- All patients should be advised about general vascular prevention measures, including BP and cholesterol reduction, stopping smoking, and starting aspirin.
- Patients with a tight symptomatic stenosis should be offered endarterectomy.
- Patients in atrial fibrillation should be counselled on the risks and benefits of anticoagulation (instead of aspirin).
- Management of comorbid diseases should be optimized, and an achievable drug regimen agreed.

Preventing subarachnoid haemorrhage

- The key intervention (clipping or coiling the aneurysm) is designed to prevent rebleeding.
- With conservative management, rebleeding after 3 months occurs at about 3% a year.
- Control of high BP and stopping smoking are epidemiologically sensible if unproven by trial.
- People with two or more first or second degree relatives with SAH are at increased risk (especially if there are two first degree relatives, including a sibling). They may be considered for MRA screening, although there is no proven benefit from this approach.
- Intervening on asymptomatic aneurysms, detected during angiography after a bleed, or during imaging for another purpose (e.g. endarterectomy), or because of screening of relatives, depends on the circumstances (Box 10.12).

Box 10.12 Risk of rupture of asymptomatic aneurysms

A cohort of 4060 patients with unruptured intracranial aneurysms was followed up for up to 6 years: 1692 did not have aneurysm repair, 1917 had surgery, and 451 had endovascular treatment.

No history of subarachnoid haemorrhage (n = 1077)

- 5-year risk of rupture for anterior circulation aneurysms (internal carotid, anterior communicating, anterior or middle cerebral arteries) was:
  - 0 for aneurysms under 7 mm
  - 2.6% for aneurysms 7–12 mm
  - 14.5% for aneurysms 13–24 mm
  - 40% for aneurysms over 25 mm.
- 5-year risk of rupture for posterior circulation aneurysms (including posterior communicating arteries) was:
  - 2.5% for aneurysms under 7 mm
  - 14.5% for aneurysms 7–12 mm
  - 18.4% for aneurysms 13–24 mm
  - 50% for aneurysms over 25 mm.
- Cavernous sinus carotid aneurysms were at less risk of rupture (0, 0, 3%, and 6% by size, over 5 years).
- The paradox is that small aneurysms are much more common than larger ones, so 60% of ruptured aneurysms are <5 mm.

Patients with a history of subarachnoid haemorrhage (from another aneurysm; n = 615)

Risk of rupture was similar to those without previous SAH apart from a 5-year risk of 1.5% (anterior circulation) and 3.4% (posterior circulation) for aneurysms under 7 mm.

Surgical and endovascular treatment

- 2.3% (surgery) and 3.1% (endovascular) died within a year, and 12.2% (surgery) and 9.5% (endovascular) had the combined poor outcome of death plus dependency or cognitive impairment a year after treatment.
- Age over 50 years, aneurysms over 12 mm, posterior circulation aneurysms, non-rupture symptoms (e.g. cranial nerve palsy), and previous ischaemic stroke were associated with poor outcome after open surgery.
- Aneurysms over 12 mm, and posterior circulation aneurysms, but not age, were associated with poor outcome after endovascular treatment.

Conclusions

Larger asymptomatic aneurysms are at high risk of rupture, but for most aneurysms under 12 mm the risks of surgery are as great or greater.

Lancet 2003; **362**: 103–10

Summary

1. Patients surviving a stroke are at high risk of another, and of other vascular events such as heart attacks. All should be considered for preventative interventions, but this should be tailored to the individual. Don't advise vigorous exercise to someone who cannot walk.

2. Use the principles of decision-making discussed in Chapter 6 to help decide. Give the patient options or advice, rather than telling them what to do.

3. Unless contraindicated give an antithrombotic (usually aspirin 75 mg), or anticoagulant if that is specifically indicated.

4. Reduce BP as far as feasible without causing side-effects.

5. Reduce cholesterol with a statin at maximum dose.

6. Screen for atrial fibrillation, and carotid stenosis in appropriate cases.

7. Advise smoking cessation, and refer to support services if necessary.

8. Advise weight loss, alcohol moderation, high fruit and vegetable diet, salt minimization, and regular exercise.

9. Make drug regimens feasible and as easy to take as possible. If in doubt about drug compliance settle on an achievable regimen.

10. Rapid access neurovascular or TIA clinics are an option for investigation of transient neurological episodes, and should have access to carotid duplex scanning, and give comprehensive vascular preventative advice.

11. Asymptomatic intracranial aneurysms over 12 mm diameter justify prophylactic intervention.

Outcomes and prognosis

Survival

This depends on:
- Your perspective—community or hospital.
- The type of stroke, and indicators of its severity.
- When you are making your prediction. The longer after the stroke the better the chance of surviving the episode. Half of those who die in the first month, do so within the first week.
- The age and comorbidity of the patient.

For survivors, subsequent risks of dying are about twice those of the general population:
- 2.5% a year for those under 65
- 5% per year at ages 65–74
- 10% per year over 75.

Table 11.1 Survival after stroke

		One-month mortality	One-year mortality
Where	Community	15–25%	30–35%
	Hospital	20–30%	30–40%
Type	Haemorrhage	50%	60%
	TACI	40%	60%
	PACI	4%	16%
	LACI	2%	10%
	POCI	7%	20–30%
Features	Very severe (SSS < 15)		62% (6 months)
	Severe (SSS 15–29)		34% (6 months)
	Moderate (SSS 30–44)		11% (6 months)
	Mild (SSS 45–58)		3% (6 months)

Recurrence

Cerebral infarction

Risk of recurrence is:
- 5% in a month
- 10–15% in the first year
- 5% a year after that.

These data may be pessimistic, as they were collected before the more intensive preventative regimens used nowadays, which may halve the risk.
Recurrence rates are:
- Lower in younger people (<65 years) and people with milder strokes (perhaps 3–4% per year).
- Greater in older age (>80 years), continued smoking, higher BP and atrial fibrillation.

Aetiological inference or investigation can help determine risk of recurrence:
- Patients with partial anterior circulation or posterior circulation strokes, which are often embolic, have a high risk of recurrence (17–20%) over 1 year, concentrated in the first 6 months.
- Lacunar strokes recur at the rate of 9% over 1 year, and are more evenly spread over time.

Intracerebral haemorrhage

After primary intracerebral haemorrhage recurrent strokes occur at a rate of 7% per year. Bleeds due to amyloid angiopathy are especially prone to rebleeding.

After SAH, risk of rebleeding from the culprit aneurysm without operation is very high (20% first day, 40% first month). Asymptomatic aneurysms have a 0–50% risk of bleeding over 5 years depending on their size and location (Box 10.12).

Neurological impairments and disabilities

What there is at the start, and how it changes, depends on:

- *Which population you are studying*. Hospital series tend to have worse strokes, and more impairments.
- *How carefully you look*. Sophisticated testing for neglect and sensory impairments give initial prevalences up to 80%.
- *When you look*. Early on you will include features in those who will recover or die very quickly.
- *Comorbidity*. Long follow-up of elderly populations is complicated by high death rates, recurrence, and comorbid events (such as hip fractures).
- *Mortality*. The prevalence of severe paralysis decreases with time, because of very high mortality rather than recovery (Table 11.2).

For setting goals and giving information to individual patients, it is useful to know what the chances of recovery are for a given starting point, in particular the initial severity of the problem (Tables 11.3 and 11.4).

- Useful function in the arm is unlikely if there is no return in grip after a month.
- If there is some return of arm muscle activity by a month, some large joint movement is likely to recover.
- Hand function recovers last and least.
- Arms and legs recover at about the same speed and to approximately the same extent (although the leg is slightly less often severely affected).

Table 11.2 Overall pattern of recovery of arm and leg weakness in a community stroke register, the South London Stroke Register

	Initial	3 months	1 year	2 years
Sample	1259	1259	943	295
Died	18%	37%	44%	51%
Lost	0	4%	4%	8%
Recurrence	0	3%	7%	8%
Arm				
No weakness	15%	23%	25%	22%
Mild	27%	19%	15%	10%
Moderate	10%	7%	6%	4%
Severe	20%	7%	4%	5%
Leg				
No weakness	18%	24%	28%	24%
Mild	26%	19%	13%	8%
Moderate	12%	8%	7%	5%
Severe	14%	5%	4%	4%

Data courtesy of Dr Enas Lawrence.

Table 11.3 Initial incidence and recovery from various neurological impairments

Impairment	Initially affected	Recovery and residual impairment
Arm and leg motor function	75%	80% show some recovery. Most within 3–6 weeks. Little improvement after 3 months, but some individuals improve up to a year. Flaccidity and initial severe weakness have poorer prognosis.
Hemianopia	25%	Recovers quickly if at all, mostly within 10 days. Little recovery after 28 days. 80% of complete hemianopias, and 30% of partial field losses persist (50% and 10%, respectively, die)
Visual and sensory inattention	20% each	Perhaps half recover
Sensory loss	30%	Perhaps half recover
Dysphasia	25%	Initial severe dysphasia, 50% survivors remain moderately or severely affected. Initial moderate dysphasia, 15% of survivors persist no better or worse. Initial mild dysphasia, 9% have persisting problems. Little recovery after 10 weeks.
Dysarthria	25%	Generally recovers
Cognition	25%	Initially difficult to estimate due to drowsiness or dysphasia. Some recovery may occur over 6–12 months. 10–20% have persisting problems.
Urinary incontinence	50%	A third of initially incontinent patients recover within 4 weeks. 20% of 6-month survivors are incontinent.
Faecal incontinence	30%	10% of 6-month survivors are incontinent
Walking (any assistance)	60%	64% survivors independent, 14% with assistance, 22% remain unable to walk at 6 months. Some further recovery possible between 6 and 12 months.

Table 11.4 Recovery according to initial level of function (Copenhagen Stroke Study)

Function	Initial severity	Recovery at 6 months
Arms	Mild–moderate weakness	80% good function, 20% no recovery (10% die)
	Severe weakness	17% of survivors recover good function, another 17% recover partially (40% die)
Legs	Complete paralysis	12% of survivors regain independent walking, 12% walk with assistance (56% die)
	Moderate–severe weakness (without complete paralysis)	40% of survivors regain independent walking, 20% walk with assistance (30% die)
	Mild weakness	80% of survivors regain independent walking, 10% walk with assistance (10% die)
Walking	Unable	22% of survivors eventually walk independently, 22% walk with assistance (40% die)
	With assistance	60% of survivors eventually get independent, 35% walk with assistance (5% die)
Aphasia	Mild	Reach a plateau within 2 weeks. Half recover completely, most of the rest remain mildly affected (20% die)
	Moderate	Reach a plateau within 6 weeks. Half of survivors recover completely, another 40% remain mildly affected (30% die)
	Severe	Reach a plateau within 10 weeks. A quarter of survivors recover completely, another quarter remain mildly affected (70% die)

Independence

- Half of survivors are independent in basic ADL after 6 months.
- By 1 year 60% of survivors are independent, largely because the most disabled have died, rather than real recovery. Another 20% are no more than mildly disabled.
- 20% of survivors require institutional care 1 year after their stroke.
- Prognosis for independence at one year varies by stroke subtype:
  - TACS 4% overall (10% of survivors);
  - PACS 60% overall (70% of survivors);
  - LACS 60% overall (67% of survivors);
  - POCS 60% overall (75% of survivors).
- Prognosis for independence at 1 year varies by initial neurological severity (SSS):
  - very severe (SSS <15) 4%
  - severe (SSS 15–29) 13%
  - moderate (SSS 30–44) 37%
  - mild (SSS 45–58) 68%.

Discharge

- Discharge prospects vary with initial stroke severity (Table 11.5).
- One-third of survivors of severe strokes are discharged home with no more than mild disability.

Table 11.5 Discharge destination according to initial stroke severity (Copenhagen Stroke Study)

	Died	Own home	Nursing home
Very severe (SSS < 15)	62%	23%	14%
Severe (SSS 15–29)	34%	34%	32%
Moderate (SSS 30–44)	11%	75%	14%
Mild (SSS 45–58)	3%	93%	4%

SSS, Scandinavian Stroke Scale.

Outcome of subarachnoid haemorrhage

- 25% die within 24 h.
- 50% die within 3 months.

Mortality from SAH, and dependency among the survivors, are quite high, but vary with:
- The patient's age.
- Level of consciousness at onset (Table 11.6).
- Angiographic findings (perimesencephalic better than aneurysmal; anterior better than posterior circulation).
- CT findings (perimesencephalic distribution, amount of blood, intraventricular blood).
- Focal neurological signs.

The majority of 'good grade' patients will make a good recovery. However, a few initially comatose patients will also recover well.

Table 11.6 Overall outcomes 6 months after SAH

Level of consciousness on admission	Mortality (%)	Good recovery (%)
Alert	13%	74%
Drowsy	28%	54%
Stuperose	44%	30%
Comatose	72%	11%

Journal of Neurosurgery 1990; **73**: 18–36.

Summary

1. Overall 1-month mortality after a stroke is 20–30%, and 1-year mortality 30–40%.
2. However, survival is very variable depending on age, type of stroke, and indicators of severity. Prognosis for some is very much better.
3. Stroke recurrence is 10% in the first year, 5% a year after that.
4. Survivors of stroke recover to some extent. 4% of patients with very severe strokes recover to independence, whereas 70% of mild strokes do. The majority will regain walking, independently or with assistance.
5. Overall 30–40% of patients (70% of survivors) are left with no more than mild limb weakness. There is little neurological recovery after 3 months, although functional recovery continues longer, especially for the most severely affected.
6. Between 20% (initially very severe) and 90% (initially mild) will achieve discharge home.
7. About half of SAH patients die, but most of the remainder make a good functional recovery.

Appendices

Appendices: Abbreviated Mental Test (AMT) score (each item scores 1 point)

1. Age.
2. Time (nearest hour).
3. Address (42 West Street).
4. Year.
5. Name of hospital.
6. Recognize two people.
7. Date of birth (month, year).
8. Year of First World War.
9. Name of monarch.
10. count backwards from 20 to 1.

Age and Ageing 1972; **1**: 233–8.

Appendices : Folstein Mini-Mental State Examination (MMSE)

Domain	Items	Score
Place	Immediate location (ward or clinic name); hospital, town, county, country	(5 points)
Time	Day, date, month, year, season	(5 points)
Registration	Repeat three objects (e.g. 'apple, coat, table')	(3 points)
Concentration	spell WORLD backwards (you can introduce this by asking them to spell it forwards). Alternatively do the first five 'serial sevens': 100, 93, 86, 79, 72, 65	(5 points)
Recall	Recall the three objects	(3 points)
Naming	Name two objects easily at hand (e.g. pen, watch)	(2 points)
Repetition	'No ifs, ands or buts' (exactly)	(1 point)
Three-stage command	'Take this paper in your right hand, fold it in two and put it on the floor'	(3 points)
Reading	Read the following and do it 'CLOSE YOUR EYES'	(1 point)
Writing	Write a sentence (requires a subject and a verb)	(1 point)
Copy design	Intersecting pentagons	(1 point)

Journal of Psychiatric Research 1975; **12**: 189–98.

Appendices : Glasgow coma scale

Best eye opening

E1 none
E2 to pain
E3 to voice
E4 spontaneously with blinking.

Best motor response in unaffected limb

M1 no response to pain
M2 arm extension to pain (decerebrate posturing)
M3 arm flexion to pain (decorticate posturing)
M4 arm withdraws from pain
M5 hand localizes pain
M6 obeys commands.

Best verbal response

V1 none
V2 sounds, no recognizable words
V3 inappropriate words
V4 confused speech
V5 normal, orientated.

Lancet 1974; **ii**: 81.

Appendices : Days 1–3 nursing care pathway for stroke

Assessment	Action
Airway maintained	*If no*: recovery position, suction, oral airway *If maintaining own airway*: remove oral airway. Encourage coughing/chest physiotherapy
Check blood glucose	Inform doctor if initial level <3 or >10 mmol/l. Monitor 1–2 hourly if on insulin sliding scale. Pre-meal and pre-bed if on other insulin regimen
Monitor oxygen saturation	Administer oxygen to keep SaO_2 >95%. Monitor 4 hourly
Temperature >37.5°C	Inform doctor. Give regular paracetamol. Obtain sputum and urine specimens. Monitor 4 hourly
Systolic BP <140 or >200 mmHg	Inform doctor. Assess conscious level and pain. Monitor 4 hourly
Pressure sore risk assessment	Appropriate pressure mattress/turning regimen
Record SSS	*If fallen >5*: inform doctor. Decide monitoring frequency (twice daily unless informed otherwise)
Record Glasgow Coma Scale	*If fallen >2*: inform doctor. Decide monitoring frequency (hourly 4 hourly unless informed otherwise)
Swallow safe	*If failed three screens*: refer speech and language therapy. Continue nil by mouth, IV fluids. Consider nasogastric tube. Review route for medication Fluid balance chart. Mouth care. Discuss/review daily *If safe*: free fluids, normal diet
Altered diet required	Food chart. Dietician referral
IV cannula	Check site
Understanding of diagnosis	Discuss. Information booklets
Moving and handling assessment, positioning plan	Allow to transfer or walk if clearly safe. Hoist if transfers unsafe. Neurological positioning. Refer physiotherapy. Assess need for bed rails (cot sides)
Antiembolic stockings required	Check foot pulses/ankle-brachial pressure index. Measure legs. Review comfort and fit. Remove daily, check and wash legs
Continent of urine	*If no*: review, or complete assessment (urinalysis, postvoid urinary residual volume bladder scan, 48 h output chart). Consider prompted voiding. Containment plan

Assessment	Action
Continent of faeces	*If no:* review, or complete assessment (rectal exam, bowel chart, specimen if diarrhoea). Containment plan
Communication problems	*If yes:* review. speech and language therapy referral if not too drowsy. Explain to relatives
Able to dress independently	*If no:* assist. Refer occupational therapy
Disability assessment	Prestroke and admission Barthel index
Unable to sleep	*If yes:* assess why. Check position in bed. Check for pain and urinary symptoms. Medical assessment
Pain	*If yes:* assess, monitor. Give prescribed analgesics. Medical assessment
Is early discharge possible?	*If yes:* discuss with patient and family. Discuss with multidisciplinary team. Liaise with community rehabilitation service if needed

SaO₂, oxygen saturation.

Appendices: Thrombolysis work-up

- Cardiorespiratory assessment and resuscitation (adequate oxygenation, control of tachyarrhythmias and seizures, fluids for hypotension).
- History, examination, including NIH stroke scale (15 min maximum).
- Send blood urgently for clotting (prothrombin time/INR, APTT), blood count, urea and electrolytes, glucose, group and save. Urine for pregnancy test on women in whom pregnancy is possible.
- Arrange head scan.
- Monitor BP every 15 min.
- Complete suitability checklist (Appendix 6).
- Consent (or assessment of best interests). Prewritten information sheet. Document discussions.

Appendices: Suitability checklist for thrombolysis

Item	Criterion	Check
Onset	Time of onset known (time last known to be neurologically normal, time of first symptoms if subsequent progression, previous night if stroke present on waking up)	☐
Timing	Commencement of tPA infusion possible within 3 h	☐

Item	Criterion	Check
Contraindications	Age within range 18–80 years	☐
	No history of severe uncontrolled hypertension	☐
	No bleeding disorder, including:	
	no oral anticoagulants	☐
	INR < 1.4	☐
	no treatment-dose LMWH within 24 h	☐
	APTT normal if heparin within previous 48 h	☐
	platelet count > 100×10^9/l	☐
	Blood sugar within range 2.8–22.2 mmol/l	☐
	No major surgery, bleeding, or trauma in past 14 days	☐
	No previous ischaemic stroke or head injury within 3 months (excluding TIA with full recovery)	☐
	No history of any previous stroke if diabetic	☐
	No history of intracranial haemorrhage ever, including SAH, or symptoms of SAH even if CT normal	☐
	No history of structural CNS (including spinal) disease or surgery, including tumours, aneurysms or arteriovenous malformations	☐
	No diabetic retinopathy with new vessels	☐
	No peptic ulcer within past 3 months, oesophageal varices, severe liver disease, acute pancreatitis	☐
	No external cardiac massage, obstetric delivery, non-compressible arterial puncture, lumbar puncture, or biopsies within 10 days (but not menstruation)	☐
	No endocarditis or pericarditis	☐
	No cancer with increased bleeding risk	☐
	Systolic BP < 185 and diastolic < 110 mmHg	☐
	Pregnancy not possible (or pregnancy test negative)	☐
Stroke work-up	No seizure at onset	☐
	Neurological deficit present at least 30 min	☐
	Neurological deficit not minor or rapidly improving	☐
	Not severe stroke (coma, NIH score >25)	☐
	Head scan performed and reported	☐
	No intracranial bleeding on head scan	☐
	Ischaemic stroke confirmed as likely diagnosis (mimics and bleeding excluded)	☐
Consent	Consent given (or assessment of best interests made). Information sheet given.	☐
Monitoring	High dependency bed available	☐

Appendices: Monitoring schedule for thrombolysis

Restrictions

- Bed rest for 24 h.
- No urinary catheterization until at least 30 min after infusion ends.
- Avoid nasogastric tube for 24 h.
- No central venous access, arterial puncture or intramuscular injections for 24 h (except adrenaline for anaphylaxis).
- Nil by mouth for 24 h except medication.
- No anticoagulants, aspirin, or non-steroidal anti-inflammatory drugs for 24 h.

Monitoring

- High dependency bed for 24 h.
- Vital signs, and neurological observations (Glasgow Coma Scale, arm/leg weakness):
  - every 15 min for 1 h before and 2 h after starting infusion
  - every 30 min for 6 h
  - hourly until 24 h after starting infusion
- Confirm neurological deterioration by repeating full NIHSS (deterioration is ≥ 4 points).
- Arrange a CT immediately if there is neurological deterioration.
- Arrange a follow up CT after 24–36 h, before aspirin or anticoagulants are given.

Intervention

- BP—maintain below 185 mmHg systolic and 110 mmHg diastolic using IV drugs for 24 h (labetalol 10 mg IV over 2 min then 10–20 mg every 10–15 min up to maximum 150 mg; stop when response adequate).
- Look for overt bleeding and give more IV fluids if BP drops below 140/80.
- Anaphylactoid reactions may occur (in 1.5%; hypotension, bronchospasm, urticaria, rash, angio-oedema). Stop tPA infusion. Continue oxygen, give more IV fluids, chlorpheniramine (chlorphenamine) 10 mg IV, hydrocortisone 200 mg IV. If severe breathing problems or hypotension give adrenaline (500 μg = 0.5 ml of 1/1000 solution IM, repeated if necessary every 5 min).
- If level of consciousness or symptoms worsen, new headache or vomiting, or acute BP rise, stop tPA infusion. Repeat CT head scan immediately. Check FBC, fibrinogen, and clotting. Consult a haematologist urgently. Give fibrinogen concentrate (or cryoprecipitate), and platelets, if $<100 \times 10^9/l$.
- Skin, gum, and nose bleeding usually do not require action.
- If other bleeding occurs, stop tPA infusion. Most patients can be managed with fluid replacement. If deterioration continues, continue fluid resuscitation, give fibrinogen/cryoprecipitate, fresh frozen plasma/prothrombin complex concentrate, and platelets on the advice of a haematologist. Check clotting and fibrinogen after each administration, target fibrinogen 1–2 g/l.

Appendices: NIH stroke scale

Detailed administration guidelines available at http://www.ninds.nih.gov/doctors/NIH_Stroke_Scale.pdf

Function	Score	Description
Level of consciousness responsiveness	0	Fully alert, immediately responsive
	1	Drowsy, arouses to voice or shaking, and responds appropriately
	2	Stuporous; aroused with difficulty; needs painful stimulus; lapses back when unstimulated
	3	Comatose, unresponsive to all stimuli
LOC orientation	0	Knows own age, and correct month *on initial answer. No coaching.*
	1	Answers one question correctly (or intubated, severely dysarthric or language barrier)
	2	Unable to answer either question (including aphasic and stuporous patients).
LOC commands	0	Opens/closes (non-paretic) hand, and closes/opens eyes to command
	1	Does one correctly
	2	Does neither correctly
Best gaze	0	Normal
	1	Partial gaze palsy (overcome by voluntary or reflex movement)
	2	Forced deviation; total gaze paresis not overcome by oculocephalic (doll's eyes) manoeuvre
Visual fields	0	Normal (upper and lower quadrants)
	1	Partial hemianopia/quadrantanopia
	2	Complete hemianopia
	3	Bilateral hemianopia (or blind from any cause)
Facial palsy	0	Normal
	1	Minor asymmetry with smiling and speech, but good volitional movement
	2	Partial: definite weakness but some movement remains
	3	Complete (including comatose, bilateral and lower motor neurone weakness)

Appendix 8: *Continued*

Function	Score	Description
Right arm—test for drift at 90° for 10 s (count out loud)	0	No drift
	1	Drift; some fluttering
	2	Some effort against gravity but unable to keep arm up for all 10 s
	3	No effort against gravity but muscle movement present
	4	No movement
Left arm	0	No drift
	1	Drift; some fluttering
	2	Some effort against gravity but unable to keep arm up for all 10 s
	3	No effort against gravity but muscle movement present
	4	No movement
Right leg—test lifting to 30° for 5 s (count out loud)	0	No drift
	1	Drift; some fluttering
	2	Some effort against gravity but unable to keep arm up for all 5 s
	3	No effort against gravity but muscle movement present
	4	No movement
Left leg	0	No drift
	1	Drift; some fluttering
	2	Some effort against gravity but unable to keep arm up for all 5 s
	3	No effort against gravity but muscle movement present
	4	No movement
Limb ataxia (out of proportion to weakness)	0	Normal (finger–nose and heel–shin tests) or too weak to test
	1	Present unilaterally in either arm or leg
	2	Present unilaterally in both arm and leg, or bilaterally

Function	Score	Description
Sensory—tested with pin/pain (not hands or feet)	0	Normal
	1	Mild: pinprick less sharp, patient aware of being tested
	2	Severe: patient unaware of being tested (including coma)
Language—aphasia testing (naming, describing picture)	0	Normal language
	1	Mild to moderate aphasia; word finding errors, naming errors, paraphrasias, mild impairment of communication either by comprehension or expression disability
	2	Severe aphasia: fully developed expressive or receptive aphasia
	3	Mute or global aphasia (or coma)
Dysarthria (give sentence list)	0	Normal articulation
	1	Mild to moderate dysarthria: patient has problems with articulation with mild to moderate slurring of words. The patient can be understood
	2	Near unintelligible or worse (or mute or unresponsive)
Neglect—testing the ability to recognize simultaneous stimuli of sensation and vision	0	No neglect; can recognize double sensory cutaneous stimulation and able to identify images in both visual fields simultaneously
	1	Partial neglect: unable to recognize both stimuli simultaneously for either cutaneous or visual
	2	Complete neglect: unable to recognize both stimuli for both cutaneous and visual

Appendices: Scandinavian Stroke Scale

Function	Score	Description
Consciousness	6	Fully conscious
	4	Somnolent, can be awaked to full consciousness
	2	Reacts to verbal command, but is not fully conscious
	0	Unresponsive to verbal command
Eye movement	4	No gaze palsy
	2	Gaze palsy present
	0	Conjugate eye deviation
Arm, motor power, affected side	6	Raises arm with normal strength
	5	Raises arm with reduced strength
	4	Raises arm with flexion in elbow
	2	Can move, but not against gravity
	0	Paralysis
Hand, motor power, affected side	6	Normal strength
	4	Reduced strength in full range
	2	Some movement, fingertips do not reach palm
	0	Paralysis
Leg, motor power, affected side	6	Normal strength
	5	Raises straight leg with reduced strength
	4	Raises leg with flexion of knee
	2	Can move, but not against gravity
	0	Paralysis
Orientation	6	Correct for time, place, and person
	4	Two of these
	2	One of these
	0	Completely disorientated
Speech	10	No aphasia
	6	Limited vocabulary or incoherent speech
	3	More than yes/no but not longer sentences
	0	Only yes/no or less
Facial palsy	2	None/dubious
	0	Present

Function	Score	Description
Gait	12	Walks 5m without aids
	9	Walks with aids
	6	Walks with help of another person
	3	Sits without support
	0	Bedridden/wheelchair

Appendices: Care pathway for urinary continence assessment and management

1. Complete within a week of admission.
2. Document history of continence problems and lower urinary tract symptoms (urgency, frequency, dysuria, nocturia, poor stream, hesitancy).
3. Consider non-bladder factors which may affect continence:
   - functional
     - mobility
     - dysphasia
     - language
     - spatial relations
     - drowsiness
     - dementia or delirium
     - dexterity
   - environmental
     - distance to toilet
     - privacy
     - ability to reach aid
     - equipment available
     - staff available
   - behavioural
     - current medication
     - ability to recognize cues
     - ability to recognize toilet
     - inhibitions
     - depression
     - motivation.
4. Commence 48-h fluid balance/frequency-volume chart. Identify functional bladder capacity (largest void), number of voids day/night, total volume passed day/night.
5. Urinalysis, and culture if positive.
6. Exclude incomplete bladder emptying (bladder scan) and faecal impaction.
7. Identify diagnoses.
   - faecal impaction (laxatives);
   - urinary infection (antibiotics, cranberry juice, avoid catheter, exclude incomplete emptying, image upper urinary tracts if male or recurrent, topical oestrogen);
   - nocturnal polyuria (check glycosuria, calcium, oedema, heart failure, renal function, consider daytime diuretics or desmopressin);
   - bladder instability (increase fluids, reduce caffeine, bladder training, pelvic floor exercises, anticholinergic drugs);
   - stress incontinence (pelvic floor exercises, cones, electrotherapy, biofeedback);
   - outflow obstruction—consider benign prostatic hyperplasia or carcinoma, stricture (alpha-blocker, finasteride, refer urology);
   - hypocontractility (stop anticholinergic drugs, try alpha-blocker, bladder stimulator, intermittent catheter, indwelling catheter);
   - drug side-effects (review diuretics, anticholinergic drugs);
   - atrophic urethritis (topical oestrogen).
8. Consider prompted voiding ('regular toileting').
9. Optimize containment—pads, sheath catheter.

Appendices: Rivermead Motor Assessment. Each item is scored 1 (succeed) or 0 (fail)

- Sit, feet unsupported 10 s
- Lying to sitting on side of bed
- Sit to standing in 15 s for 15 s
- Transfer from chair to chair towards unaffected side
- Transfer from chair to chair towards affected side
- Walk 10 m independently with an aid
- Climb stairs, may use a banister
- Walk 10 m independently without an aid
- Walk 5 m, pick up a bean bag from floor and return
- Walk outside 40 m (with aid if required)
- Walk up and down four steps (no banister or wall support)
- Run 10 m in 4 s
- Hop on affected leg five times on the spot

Appendices: The Barthel Index

Activity	Criterion	Score
Continence of urine	Continent	2
	Wet less than once a day	1
	Wet once a day or more, or catheter	0
Continence of faeces	Continent	2
	Soils less than once a week	1
	Soils more than once a week (or given enemas)	0
Toilet use	Independent (including clothes and wiping)	2
	Needs some help	1
	Unable or full help	0
Transfers (bed–chair)	Independent	3
	Minor help (help of one)	2
	Major help (can sit, needs one or two)	1
	Unable (cannot stand)	0
Walking (on the flat, using any aid)	Independent (at least 10 m)	3
	Needs human help	2
	Wheelchair independent (including round corners)	1
	Unable	0
Feeding	Independent	2
	Help cutting up, buttering bread	1
	Unable	0
Dressing	Independent (including buttons, zips, laces)	2
	Manages half	1
	Unable	0
Grooming (teeth, hair, shaving, wash face)	Independent	1
	Needs help	0
Using bath or shower	Independent	1
	Needs help	0
Stairs	Independent	2
	Needs help (verbal/physical/carrying aid)	1
	Unable	0

Appendices: Framingham risk scores, for people not in atrial fibrillation

Risk score	Points 0	+ 1	+ 2	+ 3	+ 4	+ 5	+ 6	+ 7	+ 8	+ 9	+ 10
Risk score for men aged 55–85 years											
Age (years)	54–56	57–59	60–62	63–65	66–68	69–72	73–75	76–78	79–81	82–84	85
Untreated systolic BP (mmHg)	97–105	106–115	116–125	126–135	136–145	146–155	156–165	166–175	176–185	186–195	196–205
Treated systolic BP (mmHg)	97–105	106–112	113–117	118–123	124–129	130–135	136–142	143–150	151–161	162–176	177–205
Diabetes	No		Yes								
Current smoker	No			Yes							
CVD	No				Yes						
ECG LVH	No					Yes					

Stroke 1994; **25**: 40–3.

Risk score	Points 0	+1	+2	+3	+4	+5	+6	+7	+8	+9	+10
Risk score for women aged 55–85 years											
Age (years)	54–56	57–59	60–62	63–64	65–67	68–70	71–73	74–76	77–78	79–81	82–84
Untreated systolic BP (mmHg)	95–106	107–118	119–130	131–143	144–155	156–167	168–180	181–192	193–204	205–216	
Treated systolic BP (mmHg)	95–106	107–113	114–119	120–125	126–131	132–139	140–148	149–160	161–204	205–216	
Diabetes	No			Yes							
Cigarettes	No			Yes							
CVD	No		Yes								
ECG LVH	No				Yes						

CVD, cardiovascular disease (history of MI, angina, intermittent claudication, heart failure); ECG LVH left ventricular hypertrophy on electrocardiography.

Conversion of points from risk factor profiles to probability of stroke over 10 years

Points	10-year probability (%), men	10-year probability (%), women	Points	10-year probability (%), men	10-year probability (%), women	Points	10-year probability (%), men	10-year probability (%), women
1	3	1	11	11	8	21	42	43
2	3	1	12	13	9	22	47	50
3	4	2	13	15	11	23	52	57
4	4	2	14	14	13	24	57	64
5	5	2	15	20	16	25	63	71
6	5	3	16	22	19	26	68	78
7	6	4	17	26	23	27	74	84
8	7	4	18	29	27	28	79	
9	8	5	19	33	32	29	84	
10	10	6	20	37	37	30	88	

Appendices: Risk of stroke in people with atrial fibrillation

(Excluding rheumatic mitral stenosis, who should all be considered at high risk; people on warfarin; and people within 30 days of going into atrial fibrillation.) *JAMA* 2003; **290**: 1049–56. Excel spreadsheet available at http://www.nhlbi.nih.gov/about/framingham/stroke.htm.

Conversion of points derived from risk factor profile to probability of stroke over 5 years

Points	5-year probability (%)	Points	5-year probability (%)	Points	5-year probability (%)
0–1	5	13	18	23	44
2–3	6	14	19	24	48
4	7	15	21	25	51
5	8	16	24	26	55
6–7	9	17	26	27	59
8	11	18	28	28	63
9	12	19	31	29	67
10	13	20	34	30	71
11	14	21	37	31	75
12	16	22	41		

Risk score	Points										
	0	+1	+2	+3	+4	+5	+6	+7	+8	+9	+10
Age (years)	54–59	60–62	63–66	67–71	72–74	75–77	78–81	82–85	86–90	91–93	>93
Sex	Male						Female				
Systolic BP (mmHg)	<120	120–139	140–159	160–179	>179						
Diabetes	No		Yes								
Prior stroke or TIA	No			Yes							

Index